REVERSING
HASHIMOTO'S

A 3-Step Process for Losing Weight,
Ending Fatigue and Reducing Brain Fog

ANSHUL GUPTA, MD

REVERSING HASHIMOTO'S

A 3-Step Process for Losing Weight, Ending Fatigue and Reducing Brain Fog

Design by
Transcendent Publishing
PO Box 66202
St. Pete Beach, FL 33736
www.TranscendentPublishing.com

ISBN: 978-1-7374553-4-9

This book is not intended to diagnose, treat, cure, or prevent any disease and is not intended to be the medical advice of a physician. The reader should regularly consult a physician in matters relating to his/her health and particularly with respect to any symptoms that may require diagnosis or medical attention. The use of this book implies your acceptance of this disclaimer.

Printed in the United States of America.

DEDICATION

To my mom and dad for inspiring me.

My wife, Kanwal, for being my rock,
and to my lovely kids, Nirvaan and Siya.

And to all people with Hashimoto's
who are trying to find answers.

CONTENTS

FOREWORD

by Terry Wahls, MD

Many patients wish their doctors could understand their plight. Through his own healing journey, Dr. Anshul Gupta was "gifted" with this insight early on, making him a more compassionate and empathetic physician. Now, in addition to his groundbreaking Hashimoto's work, he is on a mission to help one million people reverse their health conditions. Dr. Gupta's mission is to transform the care of Hashimoto's patients through his blog, videos, virtual Functional Medicine practice, and now this book, *Reversing Hashimoto's*.

Hashimoto's disease affects more than fourteen million people in the United States alone; however, it remains highly misunderstood by the traditional medical community. Though Hashimoto's exists under the umbrella of "thyroiditis," and its symptoms often mirror those of other thyroid conditions, it has nuances that can make it particularly difficult to treat. Indeed, there is currently only one recognized course of action prescribed to these patients, which unfortunately does not address the root cause. As a result, most Hashimoto's patients continue to experience symptoms, from weight gain and fatigue to memory loss and muscle pain. When they tell their doctors about their fatigue, memory loss, muscle pain, or weight gain, the symptoms are often dismissed as not related to Hashimoto's. Nothing helps, and many slip into hopelessness.

Dr. Anshul Gupta, speaker, author, researcher, and global expert in Hashimoto's disease, knows this journey well. As a young physician in his mid-thirties, he went through his own struggle with a seemingly untreatable illness. After seeing several specialists, he continued to experience a worsening of his symptoms that drained him of his energy and joy for living. No one could explain what was happening to his body, and in fact, he was advised to seek psychiatric help, which left him feeling alone and foolish even though he is a physician. This experience motivated him to embark on his own search for healing, and he discovered a combination of nutrition and stress-relieving techniques that not only completely cured his symptoms but led him to better physical and mental health than ever before.

Vowing that his patients would never feel that sense of hopelessness, Dr. Gupta pursued an advanced certification in Functional Medicine, which focuses on finding and treating the root causes of disease rather than merely the symptoms. This is achieved by examining the interrelation of the various systems of the body and their impact on one's overall physical and mental wellbeing. He soon found his practice flooded with patients who were experiencing the same desperation he had felt during his own health crisis. They too had made the rounds of specialists; they too had been given multiple pharmaceuticals treatments with little to no success; they too had been told to "be patient" or, much more distressing, that they would just have to learn to "live with it." Many of them, he noticed, had thyroid disorders, specifically Hashimoto's, which motivated him to begin a deep dive into the causes of this mysterious and all-too-common autoimmune disease.

This search yielded answers that were both surprising and startlingly simple. Our bodies, specifically our highly delicate thyroid glands, are being assaulted daily by a myriad of toxins in our environment, including chemicals and other substances in our foods and homes. This, coupled with nutritional choices and our stressful modern lives, is damaging to the connection between our thyroid and cellular function, specifically that of our mitochondria. The role of impaired mitochondria in the development of various autoimmune diseases is well-known; however, relatively few researchers have focused on the nexus between mitochondrial dysfunction and Hashimoto's. Even fewer have written about it in a way that patients can understand and implement themselves.

Reversing Hashimoto's is the result of that research. It steps out of the box to look at this debilitating disease through a new lens. This is a roadmap for creating health. Dr. Gupta draws on numerous studies, as well as his work at Cleveland Clinic and the success stories of the thousands of patients he has helped to overcome their health challenges and feel better than they have in years. In *Reversing Hashimoto's,* he reveals his practical, common sense three-step program that will revolutionize the treatment of this disease. If you have Hashimoto's, regardless of your circumstances and the severity of your symptoms, *Reversing Hashimoto's* can transform your life.

INTRODUCTION

H ave you ever felt scared or hopeless due to a health crisis? If so, I understand exactly where you are coming from.

I felt both of these emotions when I was just thirty-two years old and suffering from significant health problems for which nobody had answers.

This all started after I finished my Family Medicine residency and started working as a primary care physician in rural Virginia. It was a dream job for me – the practice was located in a very nice close-knit community in close proximity to nature, and I had a great team of colleagues. Above all, I felt a sense of purpose in being able to serve the people who needed my help the most.

Just two years into my career I started experiencing some mysterious symptoms. I had stomach pain and put on some weight; my mental clarity was drastically reduced by the evening, and I was fatigued all the time.

Initially, I ignored these symptoms and kept pushing forward. To be honest, I didn't even realize these *were* symptoms, as my conventionally-trained mind did not recognize things like reduced mental clarity or fatigue as real issues.

When the weight gain continued and the stomach pain became a daily occurrence, I started to become alarmed. Being a physician, I treated myself with medications for my stomach, but that didn't work. On a couple of occasions my stomach pain was so severe that I thought about going to the ER, but having worked in an ER myself I knew they would likely just give me pain medications that would not address the real problem. Something else was going on.

Finally, I made an appointment with a Gastroenterologist, who suggested doing an endoscopy and blood tests, as well as some advanced tests. Though this seemed like a very serious move to me, I felt I had no choice but to go ahead with the tests.

The tests all came back normal except for a small hiatal hernia. The Gastroenterologist added more medications to what I was already taking, but they made no difference and I continued to suffer. In fact, my symptoms were getting worse and my concern was growing. What was wrong with me?

Next, I went to see an allergy specialist to find out if I was allergic to any foods I was eating. That doctor, in the first five minutes of the appointment, declared that my issues were caused by depression and stress and I should see a psychiatrist. I was taken aback by this, because I didn't feel depressed at all; in fact, I felt like I was living my life to the fullest. The only thing that was "depressing" was my health concerns! That devastating visit left me feeling lonely, scared, hopeless, and even stupid for going to these different doctors and sharing my story with them. At the time, it seemed like I might have to live this way for the rest of my life.

That fear and desperation led me to shift my mindset. Logically, I knew the answer had to be out there – it just hadn't been found yet. I started investigating on my own, and that's when I discovered Functional Medicine. It quickly became apparent to me that Functional Medicine looked at diseases through a totally different lens from what I was used to; namely, it focused on the root cause(s) of an issue rather than just the symptoms. I also found many case studies in which physicians practicing Functional Medicine helped people with similar problems get better. Truthfully, just knowing there were others out there in the same situation was a huge relief. I also started to feel hope that I too might regain my health.

I got some training in Functional Medicine and started applying it in my own life. The first big a-ha moment for me was that my diet was very poor and was full of foods that cause inflammation. I stopped eating those foods and started eating more vegetables and good fats. I also figured out that I was sensitive to dairy, gluten, fried food, alcohol, and soy. The toughest part was giving up dairy because I love cheese, but whenever I "cheated" my gut symptoms immediately got worse. Finally, I gave up dairy and saw phenomenal results. (I did try several kinds of dairy-free cheese but they all tasted like cardboard to me).

The green smoothies I started having in the morning were also a game-changer. At first my colleagues at the clinic would take one look at my smoothie and tell me it looked awful. But once they tried it, they realized it was not so bad.

In additional to the nutritional changes I started doing some yoga, both for daily exercise and to reduce stress. I also started a simple meditation practice. Within a month of starting this program, my stomach pain was gone. Literally *gone*. Within six months, I was off all medications, had lost forty pounds, and was full of energy and focus. Even more incredible, the eczema and allergies I'd had since childhood got better too. I had not only gotten my life back – it was even better than before!

Though I had experienced it firsthand, it was sometimes hard to believe that these simple lifestyle changes could have such a profound effect on my health and wellbeing. But I couldn't deny how good I felt, or that in a very short time I had gone from hopelessness to a renewed sense of joy and power. As a physician, I had a new mission: to help my patients use functional medicine tools to shift their own health. I also made a promise to myself that I would never let anyone feel the way I had felt when there was nobody to help me.

Later on, while working at Cleveland Clinic Functional Medicine Department, I saw patients with Hashimoto's disease who had been through a similar ordeal. They had seen several doctors, and despite following medical advice and taking the prescribed medications they were still suffering with fatigue, weight problems, stomach issues, and brain fog. The worst part was the fear that they would have to live this way forever.

Like me, they all had lost hope. Not only had they been told there was nothing else that could be done; in many cases, they had also been told the lack of improvement was their fault, that they should be stricter with their diets or do more exercise. Nobody took the time to listen to their symptoms and figure out what was really going on.

After hearing their stories, I knew I had to do something to help people suffering from Hashimoto's. As I did in my own case, I launched an investigation into the disease, then started implementing my findings with my Hashimoto's patients.

The results were phenomenal. Not only did these patients experience significant improvement in their symptoms, their lab work improved as well. This was so surprising to some of the conventional doctors that they had one of my patients repeat the bloodwork to confirm that her Hashimoto's antibodies had returned to normal. The Endocrinologist had never seen anything like it and thought it was a lab error! Indeed, when the repeated lab work showed normal thyroid numbers, he was at a loss for words.

Since that time I have helped thousands of patients to regain their health and go from hopeless and helpless to empowered and in control of their disease. Now, instead of suffering from dreadful symptoms daily, they are living life to the fullest.

In this book, I will share with you exactly what I found through my work with Hashimoto's patients, including the real reason they are not getting better with conventional medicine. I also share my three-step process to help you reverse Hashimoto's and get your life back.

My goal is for every person suffering from Hashimoto's to know that there is hope and there is no reason for them to suffer any longer.

PART I

CHAPTER 1

THE REAL REASON HASHIMOTO'S PATIENTS ARE NOT FEELING BETTER

After taking care of Hashimoto's patients for several years, I realized that we are looking at this disease in a totally wrong way.

Currently, the only conventional treatment available for Hashimoto's patients is to prescribe levothyroxine, which often does not bring relief from the symptoms. Why is this? Because conventional thinking is that Hashimoto's is caused by a deficiency of thyroid hormone, which is absolutely not the case.

Hashimoto's is an *autoimmune disease*, which means the patient's immune system is producing antibodies against their own bodies, especially their thyroid gland.

These antibodies start destroying your thyroid gland until it is unable to produce enough thyroid hormone to keep up with the demand of the body. This is when patients are typically started on levothyroxine.

Unfortunately, there is no conventional medicine to stop these antibodies, so the destruction of the thyroid gland continues in spite of the thyroid medications. So you see, when doctors try to treat Hashimoto's with levothyroxine, they're not treating the real problem (antibody production); they're simply replenishing the reduced thyroid hormone, which has resulted from the destruction caused by these antibodies.

This is precisely the reason patients with Hashimoto's continue to suffer from symptoms even while taking medication. The worst part is that after several years of having Hashimoto's most of these patients also develop other autoimmune diseases like Rheumatoid Arthritis, Lupus, et cetera. This is because the antibodies produced due to Hashimoto's also affect other body parts.

As mentioned above, conventional medicine doesn't have any methods to help Hashimoto's patients reduce these antibodies. In fact, if you ask your doctor about ways to reduce antibodies, they will tell you *it can't happen*.

This is where Functional Medicine comes in. Using the concepts of Functional Medicine, I have devised a protocol to reduce these antibodies and help reverse Hashimoto's symptoms.

First, though, there is more to understand about Hashimoto's.

Most doctors believe that Hashimoto's only destroys the thyroid gland, but this is not the case. In fact, it is also responsible for the destruction of another important structure present in every cell of our body – *the mitochondria.*

Okay, so what are mitochondria? In simplest terms, mitochondria are the "powerhouse of the cell" because they are responsible for producing energy from the food we eat. However, there is much more to them than that.

New research shows that mitochondria are also responsible for controlling various metabolic processes, are involved in controlling inflammation, and play an important role in the aging process.

But the bigger question is, what has mitochondria to do with Hashimoto's disease?

My findings indicate that there is a special connection between mitochondria and thyroid. I call this the *mito-thyroid connection*.

Though conventional medicine has known about this connection for years now, it has neglected its importance with regard to Hashimoto's patients.

The mitochondria controls the optimal functioning of our body, and they take their signals from thyroid hormone. This is the reason thyroid hormone medicine alone does not work: it fixes the signal, but it does not improve the health of the machinery of the cell.

Let's try to understand this connection with a simple example.

Imagine your body is a car. Your thyroid gland is the gas pedal and your mitochondria is the engine. Under normal circumstances, when you press the gas pedal it sends a signal to the engine to work more and put out more power. Now imagine there is something damaging the engine and not letting it work properly. Then it doesn't matter how much you press the gas pedal; in fact, pressing it harder will only reduce the efficiency of the car. To get the car working again, we need to fix the engine.

This is what is happening in Hashimoto's disease. The mito-thyroid connection is broken, which leads to all the symptoms associated with it. And instead of working on restoring this connection, we keep pumping patients full of thyroid hormones. In the meantime, the patient continues to experience fatigue, weight problems, brain fog, and hair loss – all of which are manifestations of unhealthy mitochondria.

When you think about it, this makes a lot of sense. Fatigue, brain fog, and weight gain are all "lack of energy" issues, indicating the problem lies with the reduced function of the "powerhouse of the cell."

Why is the connection between thyroid and mitochondria broken in Hashimoto's?

The research shows that Hashimoto's disease happens because of the interplay between *your genetics and the environment around you.*

What this means is that your body's unique genetic makeup makes you sensitive to certain environmental factors. And once you get exposed to them, your body starts to produce antibodies which ultimately leads to the destruction of this mito-thyroid connection.

This happens in two phases:

1. Trigger phase: This is when you are exposed to an environmental factor or factors that you are sensitive

to. Everyone has different triggers, but the main culprits are certain foods, toxins, infections, stress, and nutritional insufficiencies. We will get into greater detail about them in future chapters.

When your body gets exposed to these external triggers it causes your immune system to start making antibodies against your own body. These antibodies start the destruction of this mito-thyroid connection.

2. Continuation Phase: The destruction of the mito-thyroid connection leads to the development of inflammation in the body. This inflammation is caused because of excessive production of reactive oxygen species (ROS). ROS are normally generated in mitochondria as waste products when energy is produced. As mentioned above, the main function of mitochondria is to produce energy, so ROS production happens all the time. Our bodies have an innate mechanism to get rid of these ROS; however, in those with Hashimoto's disease, this mechanism starts failing, which leads to an excessive production of ROS. This excess ROS leads to inflammation in the body, which further destroys this mito-thyroid connection.

What we have now is a never-ending cycle of destruction and the development of symptoms like fatigue, hair loss, weight problems, feeling cold, brain fog, gut symptoms, et cetera.

Research has shown that in Hashimoto's patients, the thyroid gland has an excessive accumulation of faulty mitochondria. They also indicate an excessive production of ROS.

Do you see now why taking thyroid hormones does not stop the underlying destruction of the mito-thyroid connection? This is why people with Hashimoto's continue to suffer from symptoms even after the treatment. Moreover, these symptoms get worse over time.

What we actually need is to go to the root cause of Hashimoto's and fix the problem there. This is where my three-step process comes in. But before we delve deeper into that process, I would like to talk more about the various symptoms of Hashimoto's and their relation to the mito-thyroid connection.

Your Free Gift

A **3-Day Meal Plan** with recipes to use with this book.

This free gift is a sample 3-day meal plan based on
the principles of mito-thyroid diet.
This will give you a headstart in your
thyroid healing journey.

To claim your gift, go to:
Reversinghashimotobook.com/3-day-meal-plan

CHAPTER 2

WENDY'S WEIGHT PROBLEMS

Wendy is a thirty-two-year-old female who has been battling thyroid disorder for two years now. Before being diagnosed she had experienced symptoms of low thyroid for more than five years, but according to her doctors all tests were normal.

Over that five years Wendy had gained fifty pounds, though she had not changed her diet, and was unable to lose it. She knew something was wrong with her body and kept going to her doctors in the hope that they would figure it out, but all she heard was that she needed to watch what she ate and do more exercise. After much insistence from Wendy, one doctor finally did order a blood test for thyroid disorder, but it was only a TSH test, and it too was normal. No one bothered to check her for Hashimoto's disease.

As she continued to gain weight, Wendy grew more and more desperate. She even went on a diet that called for just nine hundred calories a day. Some of the weight did come off but her overall health deteriorated. Her skin started looking like an old lady, and she had no energy. After she passed out a couple of times, her doctor advised her against such a strict diet. He also ordered more lab work, and this time it showed that her thyroid levels were very low.

When Wendy was started on levothyroxine she was hopeful that it would finally take care of all her problems. Instead, she continued to gain weight, though at a slower rate than before the medicine. She started watching what she ate again, joined a gym, and even hired a trainer, but the weight would not come off. According to her doctors, she was on the correct dosage of levothyroxine and it might just take a while. She should be patient, they said.

Two years later, Wendy still had not seen any results. She was very frustrated and was losing hope in the medical system. The weight gain had affected her confidence and mental state; she would spend hours and hours in front of the mirror looking at her body and wondering what she could do to look better. She even thought about having cosmetic surgery to remove the excess fat around her waistline, thinking that might make her look good.

Not surprisingly, this was all taking a toll on her marriage as well. She lost all interest in having sex with her husband, as she felt that she was not good enough for him, and would say she was tired or just not in the mood. Her husband was very supportive of her, but eventually they had begun to drift apart, which of course added significantly to her emotional and mental stress.

By the time Wendy came to see me she had lost all hope; in fact, she was only there because one of her friends had insisted.

Initially, she was very hesitant to share her story with me, but when I asked her what her biggest fear was she finally broke down and replied, "I'm afraid I will look this ugly for the rest of my life." I could feel her pain, especially since I had suffered with weight issues myself. I reassured her that she was not alone in her fear and that there was hope for her to lose the weight.

Most females with thyroid disorders suffer from weight issues – it is their most common complaint. And, like Wendy, they usually cannot lose this weight even after trying different diets.

Why is this happening? That is a big question for medical professionals. The traditional thinking is that thyroid hormone controls the basal metabolic rate (BMR). In simple terms, BMR is the amount of energy your body will burn when you are at rest and not doing any activity. Someone with a high BMR burns more calories without doing any work, and therefore will be able to more easily maintain a healthy weight, or lose weight with dietary changes. The assumption is that females with low thyroid have lower BMR, but if this were true they should be able to lose weight when given drugs that replace the thyroid hormone. As Wendy and many others have discovered, however, that doesn't happen.

Why is this? Well, new research suggests that the mito-thyroid connection might be playing a role in weight gain issues. Both thyroid and mitochondria are involved in energy production; they also control how you burn fat. People who are obese have a higher concentration of dysfunctional mitochondria in their bodies, particularly in fat cells called adipocytes. These adipocytes are the main reason we accumulate fat in our body, and mitochondria play an important role in regulating their function. In fact, a research study found that mice given a supplement that supports mitochondrial function had a lower obesity rate.

We have known for a long time that mitochondrial dysfunction exists in patients with a thyroid disorder. But now we are realizing that the broken mito-thyroid connection might also be the real reason for weight gain in Hashimoto's patients. Again, to help them lose this weight, we need to stop pumping them with thyroid medicine and instead focus on fixing the mito-thyroid connection.

CHAPTER 3

FORGETFUL FREIDA

Freida was a fifty-eight-year-old female who came to see me for a thyroid disorder, her main complaint being persistent brain fog. Many people with thyroid issues suffer from this, though each one describes it differently. (Interestingly, there are no brain fog symptoms listed in medical textbooks.) Freida found it difficult to put her experience into words, except to say that over the past three years she felt her mental capacity had significantly declined.

A successful entrepreneur, she now had problems recalling dealings with her clients. At meetings she made sure to write down each and every word and would go into panic mode if she forgot her pen and paper. She feared that if things continued to worsen she might even lose her business.

Brain fog was also affecting her personal life. She would forget where her conversations were going and even sometimes froze in the middle of a sentence, unable to recall what she was about to say. After friends pointed out that she asked the same questions again and again, she started cutting back on her social interactions so she wouldn't look "dumb" in front of them. Of course, this isolation wasn't good for her mental health and she was often quite lonely. To make matters worse, she tried to explain the brain fog to her friends but they couldn't relate at all. She felt she had no one to turn to.

Frieda had been to several doctors, most of whom suggested it might be due to aging. She shouldn't worry about it, they said, she should just find ways to relax and reduce her stress. But Frieda *was* worried. She knew it wasn't normal for females in their fifties to feel this way.

At the time, she had been battling thyroid issues for more than ten years and was taking levothyroxine. Initially, her main complaint was of feeling tired and also weight issues, but she didn't worry about them as much and kept pushing through. The decline in her mental capacity was a different story, and she was becoming truly frightened. It didn't help that her mother had dementia and suffered terribly in the last years of her life. Now Freida wondered, was the same thing happening to her?

She started looking for answers on her own about what brain fog was and how she could get rid of it, and this is what eventually led her to me. Her eyes literally lit up when I told her that I not only knew what brain fog was but had successfully treated many patients with it. She had thought she was the only one who had this symptom – and no surprise there, since it doesn't exist in medical textbooks! She was so happy she'd finally found someone who understood and could offer hope for improvement.

Far from being alone, Freida was just one of many middle-aged females who experience brain fog – especially those with thyroid disorder.

Many patients suffer with brain fog for a long time, sometimes years, without sharing them with their doctors. Some, like Freida, don't exactly know how to describe this symptom. Others fear they will sound "crazy" and be referred to a psychiatrist. They often question whether what they are going through is real or just in their head. Unfortunately, when they do find the courage to talk about it to their physician, they are indeed told that they are imagining it. As I can attest, this is a very scary situation to be in.

Here are some ways in which people describe their brain fog:

1. Difficulty focusing
2. Loss of short- and/or long-term memory
3. Feeling "cloudy"
4. Problems with thinking and communicating
5. "Forgetful"
6. Inability to concentrate and multitask
7. Feeling confused
8. Trouble with word-finding

These is not an exhaustive list, just some of the most common things I have heard. Some people experience a few of these symptoms; some experience all of them.

More important than finding words to describe brain fog is figuring out why people with thyroid disorders develop it in the first place. Is it because of the deficiency of thyroid hormone, or something else? And if it is a deficiency of thyroid hormone, then why doesn't it get better when we take thyroid medicine?

15

The answer is that the real reason for the brain fog is *the destruction of the mito-thyroid connection.*

We have long known that the thyroid hormone plays a role in brain development during the early childhood years. However, there are now studies indicating that the thyroid hormone also plays a role in adult brain functioning. The brain has thyroid hormone receptors through which the thyroid hormone controls brain health; this means that maintaining healthy levels of thyroid hormone is important for proper brain function.

Even more essential to brain health is the mitochondria. In fact, the brain is one of the organs with the highest concentrations of mitochondria – this, because its functions consume so much energy. Mitochondrial dysfunction, therefore, has been associated with brain aging, and there is even evidence that it plays a huge role in dementia and Alzheimer's, which have increased in frequency in recent years. In less severe cases of mitochondrial dysfunction, symptoms of brain fog result. As in the case elsewhere in the body, the destruction of mitochondria in the brain is mainly due to underlying inflammation, excessive oxidative stress, and reactive oxygen species.

In people with Hashimoto's disease the destruction of the mito- thyroid connection is mainly responsible for brain fog. Replacing the thyroid hormone takes care of one piece of the puzzle, but we still have done nothing to help with mitochondrial health. More importantly, we have not yet addressed the real reason this mito-thyroid connection was broken in the first place. In the pages that follow, we are going to learn more about the destruction of this connection and how we can repair it.

CHAPTER 4

NANCY THE NAPPING LADY

N ancy was a thirty-eight-year-old woman who had been dealing with extreme fatigue for five years. She was so tired that she had to take two naps during the day just so she could function. Two years earlier she had been diagnosed with Hashimoto's and started on levothyroxine, yet her condition had continued to worsen.

Nancy was a happily married woman with two kids. She gave up her job when she was pregnant with her first child because she wanted to be a stay-at-home mom. The fatigue started after the birth of her second child. Initially she had thought it was because she was taking care of two children, but eventually she realized something else was going on.

Nancy was nicknamed "The Napping Lady" by her family and friends because she could fall asleep anywhere. They joked about her frequent naps, but it was no laughing matter. In fact, on days when she missed one of her naps she would crash by evening, unable to function at all.

Nancy wanted to be a good mother and tried to keep up with her children, but her fatigue often stopped her from engaging in even minor physical activity. This was a sharp contrast from before her first child, when she used to run five miles each day. Now a brisk walk around her neighborhood wore her out for the rest of the day. She felt like an eighty-year-old woman, and it was affecting her emotionally and psychologically, as well as physically.

She had been to several doctors over the years, but none had been able to offer any help. They didn't even know why she was tired all the time. All her blood tests, including those for her thyroid, came back normal. Some suggested she was depressed and that that was the cause of her fatigue. She even tried anti-depressants, which actually made her tiredness worse.

When I saw Nancy for the first time, she broke down and said: "Doctor, I am not a good mother. I can't even take care of my children because I am so tired." It was very heartbreaking to see her in that situation. Being a parent myself, I could feel her pain, her concern, and her desperation for answers.

Nancy's case is far from unique. In fact, as mentioned earlier fatigue is the most common complaint that I hear from females with Hashimoto's. Levothyroxine treatment often is not able to help.

In conventional medicine, it is thought that the deficiency of thyroid hormone is responsible for fatigue in Hashimoto's patients. But, again, the real reason is the destruction of mito-thyroid connection, which is usually caused by the triggers mentioned earlier.

The reason mitochondria are called the powerhouse of the cell is because they are responsible for energy production. They turn carbohydrates and fat into ATP, a molecule that fuels our body. It has been shown that in thyroid patients, the mitochondrial function is compromised, which interferes with energy production. Several Hashimoto's patients have been diagnosed with chronic fatigue syndrome, but now the research suggests that faulty mitochondria are actually responsible for the fatigue.

Muscle biopsies in people with chronic fatigue show a high percentage of dysfunctional mitochondria, as well as high levels of reactive oxygen species. These both suggest a strong correlation between being fatigued and faulty mitochondria.

When we give Hashimoto's patients levothyroxine we are not doing anything to fix this broken connection; that's the reason they continue to feel exhausted and not able to fully participate in life.

PART II

>

TRIGGERS FOR HASHIMOTO'S.

CHAPTER 5

FOOD SENSITIVITIES

We often hear the saying, "Food is medicine," and I wholeheartedly believe it is true, both because of my own experience and those of the many patients I have helped heal through food. That said, I think there is another aspect of nutrition that we may be neglecting, and that is food sensitivity.

Food sensitivity is a condition in which our body starts developing antibodies against particular things we consume. These antibodies then start attacking our thyroid, joints, and other parts of the body.

First, these antibodies attack your digestive system, which causes what's known as "leaky gut" – or a damaged gut lining through which antibodies, viruses, and bacteria can pass. It is through leaky gut that these food antibodies enter the body and move on to destroy other parts of the body like the thyroid, joints, et cetera.

Each and every one of us has what I call genetic weak points – basically these are areas in our body that are most vulnerable to destruction by these antibodies. In many females, this genetic weak point is the mito-thyroid connection. This destruction is gradual, taking anywhere from several months to several years, until one day the thyroid gives up. That's when it finally shows up on the blood tests. Furthermore, most doctors don't check for thyroid antibodies, they just check the TSH levels, which is why so many females complain of thyroid symptoms for several years before being diagnosed with Hashimoto's.

It is important to know the difference between food sensitivities and food allergies. Food allergy is a condition where one develops an anaphylactic reaction like swelling of their body, tongue, or difficulty breathing as soon as they consume a particular food. We have known about food allergies for a long time, as the symptoms are more pronounced and easily identifiable. The most common food allergy is to peanuts, where people break out in hives or experience swelling of the face or tongue as soon as they come into contact with them.

The symptoms of food sensitivities are much more subtle, and the damage to the body is much more gradual, sometimes taking months to years. This is why most people can easily identify the foods to which they are allergic, but not those they are sensitive to. If you have any reason to suspect you have a food sensitivity you should be tested as soon as possible. We are going to talk more about how to identify food sensitivity in Chapter 11.

I am often asked by my patients why there has been an increase in food sensitivities in recent years. There are various reasons for this, but one of the important ones is that our food has dramatically changed. Everything we eat has a genetic structure, or code, which the body recognizes and knows it's safe to consume. Now, because of modern agriculture, the genetic structure of our food is changing at a rate so rapid our bodies can't keep up with it.

Simply put, we have been using technology to modify our crops to suit our needs; for example, to increase production we make them more and more resistant to pests. The result is a change in their genetic structure, which our bodies don't recognize and treat as dangerous by developing antibodies.

Along with that, we are using more and more chemicals to grow our food. All these chemicals are also detrimental to our health and lead to the development of leaky gut. When you have a leaky gut, your body develops more food sensitivities to foods; in fact, in some people it's so severe that they find themselves reacting to every food they eat. It is because of the gut destruction from chemicals and toxins.

Yet another reason is the processing of our food. The majority of our food is processed by adding additives, preservatives or colors to it. Again, these additives lead to an increase in food sensitivities.

There are research studies that have shown a correlation between certain foods and Hashimoto's disease. One such study was done on 1887 participants; they were given various categories of foods then checked for either a positive or negative association with developing antibodies for Hashimoto's. What they found was that the people who consumed more animal fats and butter had more chances of having positive antibodies for Hashimoto's disease. There was also a case study about a patient with Hashimoto's disease who had been consuming large quantities of artificial sweeteners. Once she stopped ingesting these sweeteners, her thyroid labs, including the antibodies, all came back to normal.

There are several studies that have evaluated the link between gluten and Hashimoto's disease. A 2015 study showed that there is indeed a correlation between gluten sensitivity and the development of Hashimoto's; furthermore, the majority of studies have shown improvement of symptoms and antibody levels after the participants go gluten-free.

A research study was also done on people with celiac disease – or gluten allergies – and concluded that celiac patients had higher numbers of dysfunctional mitochondria. Researchers also noted that these celiac disease patients had higher inflammation. These findings also points to how gluten allergy and sensitivity can lead to mitochondrial dysfunction. Finally, other significant studies have shown that a diet high in glycemic load or sugar leads to mitochondrial dysfunction.

As we can see here, food is a significant factor in the development of Hashimoto's disease. I cannot stress enough how important it is to identify the foods that your body has sensitivities to so you can remove them and help your thyroid heal.

CHAPTER 6

TOXINS TRIGGERING HASHIMOTO'S

We have known about environmental toxins – and their detrimental effect on our bodies – for ages. The first toxins we became aware of were heavy metals like mercury and lead; however, while we have taken these steps to remove things like lead paint from our lives, we continue to release other toxins into our environment. Indeed, it seems like every day there are new pesticides or synthetic chemicals on the market, and when you take in account all the other toxins, such as mold in our homes, it can feel impossible to get rid of them all.

Our body has innate mechanisms to handle these toxins, but this high toxin load is causing that detox system to fail. Once they enter our body most of these toxins get deposited and, over the course of time, reach levels that threaten our health. Another issue we often neglect is the cumulative effect of having all these different toxins assaulting our bodies at once. The thyroid is a fragile endocrine gland that is very sensitive to toxin exposure, and chronic exposure leads to the development of Hashimoto's.

We are now going to talk about different kinds of toxins that can affect the thyroid, especially those that destroy the mito-thyroid connection.

Heavy Metals

1. **Mercury:** Mercury is one of the metals known to be an endocrine disruptor, meaning it harms various endocrine glands, especially the thyroid. In fact, high concentrations of mercury have been found in the thyroids of people who have only been exposed to it externally. This tells us that the thyroid is especially vulnerable to mercury, and that any exposure can get deposited into the thyroid gland. Mercury exposure is more concerning for females who have Hashimoto's disease. In fact, one study on women showed a correlation between exposure to mercury and the development of thyroid antibodies; the higher the exposure, the greater the risk. Also, mercury is poisonous to mitochondria, as several studies have shown that mercury exposure leads to mitochondrial damage. Mercury causes the formation of free radicals and also leads to the depletion of a key antioxidant called glutathione. The depletion of glutathione and formation of free radicals leads to the destruction of mitochondria, which ultimately leads to the development of symptoms of fatigue, brain fog, and weight issues in Hashimoto's patients.

   While the exact mechanism of how mercury damages the thyroid is not well established, there are some theories. One is that mercury might interfere with the utilization of iodine in the thyroid and thus interferes with thyroid hormone production. Another is that mercury may inhibit the conversion of T4 hormone to T3 hormone. This is of concern because T3 hormone is the active form of thyroid hormone, so if something interferes with the conversion of T4 to T3 it can lead to a number of health problems.

The big question here is, how do we get exposed to mercury?

There are three main chemical forms of mercury:

1. Organic mercury, which is used as fungicides, herbicides, and wood preservatives; it is also present in fish and seafood.

2. Inorganic mercury, which is used for antiseptic and dermatological preparations, and even in cosmetics.

3. Elemental mercury, which is used in the production of batteries, thermometers, and fluorescent tubes, as well as in dental amalgams.

It's easy to see how we might be getting exposed to mercury on a daily basis without even knowing it. It can be in the fish we eat, the creams we put on our skin, and the tooth fillings the dentist puts in our mouth. Therefore, when investigating the cause of our health problems it makes sense to go on the assumption that mercury is present and get tested for it.

There are several ways of checking the levels of mercury in our body. The most common is through blood work, however, a urine test is preferred because mercury levels in the urine are more stable and give us a better evaluation of chronic exposure, especially when it comes to inorganic and elemental mercury. Plus, the test can be done with a home kit instead of having to go to a lab.

2. **Lead:** It is also important to find out if you have been exposed to lead. We all know that lead house paints cause significant health issues in young children. Although such paints are not used anymore, lead is still abundant in our environment and, like mercury, can lead to thyroid issues. A study done on 5,628 females found that the presence of lead in the blood increased their chances of having autoimmune thyroid disease. Another study showed that chronic exposure, even at low levels, can cause issues with the thyroid. Lead accumulates in the mitochondria and leads to their destruction. Lead also causes high levels of free radicals, which cause further mitochondrial damage.

The most common places we can get exposed to lead are:

1. Old buildings: These structures may still have lead pipes, which can affect the water we drink and bathe in. Some people think using a simple filter will take care of this issue, but in reality only special water filters take care of this problem. The other issue in old buildings can be old lead paint; for example, if people took shortcuts and painted over it rather than taking the time to scrape it away. This can still cause low levels of exposure. If you have any reason to believe there is still lead paint in your home or office, it is imperative that arrange for its removal.

2. Water: As mentioned above, the water in our homes may be exposed to lead through our pipes. There are also other ways in which our tap and well water can become contaminated with low levels of lead. Although there are safety standards in place across the country, they are not perfect, and some things still fall through the cracks. To be safe, you must get your water tested.

As in the case with mercury, a blood test is the most common way to test for lead toxicity. But again, a urine test gives us more complete information, and often a single urine sample can give us information about all the heavy metals present in our body.

Mold Toxins

One of the most common triggers for patients with thyroid issues is mold exposure. In our modern world, mold is present almost everywhere, including our homes. Also, as it is often out of sight we don't know it's there until it starts to affect our health.

For mold to grow it needs moisture, oxygen, and food, and it gets all these things in the home. There are a number of situations that can promote mold growth, such as water leaks, flooding (i.e., after a storm), and leaky roofs. Even if you have your home repaired there might still be some remaining moisture somewhere, which along with "food" like construction materials provides the perfect environment for mold to thrive. In fact, buildings that have had water damage have a higher percentage of mold spores, so it's very important to know the history of your home and get it checked if there has been water damage in the past.

As you can see, it is almost impossible to completely avoid exposure to mold, but do not be alarmed. There are an estimated 100,000 different types of mold and many of them are harmless. Others, however, are pathogenic and can cause dysfunction in our bodies. Some of the common types include:

1. Aspergillus
2. Penicillium
3. Stachybotrys
4. Fusarium
5. Myrothecium
6. Monascus
7. Histoplasma
8. Cryptococcus

These types of molds attack our bodies and produce mycotoxins, which in turn lead to thyroid disease.

Is Mold Triggering Your Thyroid Issues?

There is a body of research showing the connection between mold exposure and thyroid diseases. One study done on aspergillus exposure and development of thyroiditis found that twenty percent of people with such exposure, and who were immunocompromised, had this thyroid problem. This was important because aspergillus is a common type of mold.

Another study showed that females who were exposed to mold-infested buildings developed thyroid illness. Specifically, they were low in the active form of thyroid hormone, T3.

Mold toxins cause inflammation in our body by producing excessive amount of reactive oxygen species. This inflammation blocks certain enzymes needed for thyroid hormone production and also destroys the mitochondria. These females were treated in the traditional way, with levothyroxine (which is T4), but did not improve because the mold toxins were blocking the conversion of T4 to T3. If you are taking this medication and are still suffering from symptoms, it is a good idea to check to see if mold toxins are the culprit.

Mold exposure has also been associated with the development of antibodies, which then destroy the mitochondria. It therefore comes as no surprise that a study found that people with a history of exposure to indoor mold, mycotoxins, and water damage had elevated levels of mitochondrial antibodies. Remember, these mitochondrial antibodies are a common trigger for autoimmune diseases like Hashimoto's.

Clearly, exposure to mold can trigger for thyroid problems, so if you are still search for the cause of your symptoms it is something that needs to be looked into.

Pesticides and Herbicides

There is a huge debate currently going on about whether the chemicals we use in agricultural practices are safe or not. The industries that produce them claim they are harmless and don't cause any adverse effects. The research studies, however, often say the opposite.

33

There are several health conditions which have been associated with exposure to these pesticides and herbicide. And I believe that they are the primary cause for the rise of autoimmune conditions in recent years.

Several pesticides have adverse effects on thyroid health and damage the thyroid in different ways. They not only interfere with thyroid hormone production, but the functioning of these thyroid hormones in our body. Also, it has been seen that these pesticides lead to the development of inflammation and destruction of mitochondria, which makes the situation worse for Hashimoto's patients. It is therefore essential these patients are checked to see if these chemicals are adding to their toxic load.

Environmental Toxins

As previously mentioned, thyroid disorders, particularly Hashimoto's, have been linked to environmental triggers. It has been proposed that several environmental chemicals might have endocrine-disrupting properties and can ultimately lead to autoimmune disease development. Unfortunately, many of our modern-day "advancements" has introduced more and more these chemicals into our lives. For example:

1. **Polybrominated diphenyl ethers (PDBE)**: These are flame retardants commonly used in furniture and other things around in the house.

   Studies have shown a reduction of thyroid hormone when people are exposed to these chemicals. It has been proposed that the way these PDBE cause harm is through the destruction of our mitochondria.

The major source of PDBE is upholstered cloth furniture, but they can also be present in other sofas, pillows, et cetera. As time goes on this furniture breaks down and releases these chemicals into your home environment, especially in the dust and air you breathe in.

The use of this chemical is declining and some states in the US have even banned it altogether, but if you have older furniture it is probably already in your home. Also, not all companies follow these regulations, and furniture manufacturers outside the country are not required to comply. The same goes for mattresses, the majority of which are also treated with fire retardants. Again, the manufacturers are not using PDBE on newer mattresses, but the older mattress might still have them, as well as those manufactured in other countries.

2. **Bisphenol A (BPA).** This is another chemical with endocrine- disrupting properties. BPA is used in clear plastic bottles, water dispensers, and the linings of food cans. BPA particularly affects the levels of T4, and appears to be most dangerous to infants and children. Most frightening is that even very low levels of BPA causes inflammation which leads to the destruction of mitochondria and thus the mito-thyroid connection – making it another potential trigger for Hashimoto's.

3. **Per- and polyfluoroalkyl substances (PFAS):** The nonstick cookware that you use in the kitchen is coated with these chemicals, which have also been linked with thyroid disorders. Like BPA, they affect the production of thyroid hormones, especially T4, and thus are

a significant cause of mitochondrial destruction and the development of Hashimoto's.

Again, some of these chemicals have been banned in the US but not worldwide. In addition, the new chemicals created to replace them are very similar in chemical composition and might lead to the same health-related issues. Unfortunately, these chemicals stay in our environment for a very long time, as evidenced by the widespread presence of PFAS in drinking water, foods, food packaging materials, and other consumer products.

As you can see, there are several kinds of toxins that are in our environment which affect our mito-thyroid connection. While avoiding exposure is difficult if not impossible, we can become aware of those that cause and exacerbate Hashimoto's and take additional precautions to decrease their burden on our body.

CHAPTER 7

STRESS TRIGGERING HASHIMOTO'S

Any discussion of environmental triggers would not be complete without talking about stress. It is probably the trigger we are exposed to most and the one we often try to ignore. Stress plays a significant role in most, if not all, diseases, including those affecting the thyroid. In fact, there are even specific studies that show the correlation between stress and the development of Hashimoto's.

Let's start by defining the term "stress," as it may be broader than you think. Stress is anything that you are uncomfortable with − emotionally, mentally, physically or spiritually. These days, we seemed to be more stressed than at any other time in history − be it because of our work, personal life, health, or events in our environment.

The next step is understanding what happens to our body when it gets exposed to stress. It secretes stress hormones called cortisol and adrenaline through the adrenal glands, which are small endocrine glands that sit on top of your kidneys. The adrenals' main function is to help our body handle stress through the secretion of these hormones.

Here's a great example of how adrenaline and cortisol work to keep us safe in times of stress. Thousands of years ago, when we were living in the jungle, there were many conditions that put us in physical peril. Let's say you're walking along one day and see a tiger. Your body immediately senses the danger and activates the stress response. The adrenals secrete the hormones to prepare your body to run from the tiger. During this time your body is conserving all its energy it will need for this activity; it's also pushing all your blood to the muscles, releasing more sugar into the blood for energy, and putting you on "high alert." You start running and, fortunately, manage to escape from the tiger. Once your body senses the danger is gone, the stress response stops.

Obviously, we live under very different conditions today; however, our bodies can't differentiate between the tiger and modern-day stressors such as work pressure, family stress, financial troubles, health challenges, traffic jams, et cetera, so it initiates the same response. The problem is, we get exposed to stress constantly so the stress response never gets shut down and have a constant surge of these stress hormones. They are very beneficial during the acute stress phase (the tiger), but when their levels are high all the time they start harming our own body.

Let's focus on cortisol, as it is the one that remains high for most people. The functions of cortisol are:

- Controlling metabolism
- Controlling inflammation

- Controlling glucose metabolism
- Controlling the body's response to stress

As you can see, cortisol plays a significant role in the proper functioning of our body. But chronically elevated high levels of cortisol are harmful and can lead to the following symptoms:

- Excessive weight gain, especially around the abdomen
- Feeling anxious or "wired"
- Fatigue
- Menstrual problems
- Thin skin

These symptoms are very typical of Hashimoto's disease too. That's how we know that that stress can lead to thyroid dysfunction.

How do high cortisol levels affect the thyroid?

It has been seen that high levels of cortisol shut down the production of thyroid hormone.

This is part of that built-in defense mechanism when your body senses external stress and needs to prioritize resources for more essential functions.

Also, cortisol affects the conversion of the T4 hormone to T3, which as we have seen throughout this book leads to various symptoms of Hashimoto's.

Cortisol is also an important regulator of our immune system, and when chronically elevated it makes changes to that system which make the body more susceptible to autoimmune diseases. Specifically, it causes the secretion of chemical substances that cause inflammation, which, as we have seen, can lead to the development of Hashimoto's disease.

Stress and cortisol also have profound effects on mitochondria. This is because cortisol regulates our body's metabolism and glucose control, which is done by influencing the functioning of mitochondria.

High cortisol levels send signals to mitochondria, which leads to changes that cause mitochondrial dysfunction. High levels of stress also lead to mitochondrial DNA damage, as does the inflammation caused by high cortisol levels.

What does all of this tell us? That exposure to stress in all its forms causes the destruction of the mito-thyroid connection and ultimately leads to the development of symptoms in Hashimoto's patients.

CHAPTER 8

INFECTIONS TRIGGERING HASHIMOTO'S DISEASE

Our body gets exposed to several pathogens such as viruses, bacteria, fungus, and parasites on a daily basis. Thanks to our immune system, we are able to ward off these infections most of the time. Other times, however, these pathogens will bypass our defense system and cause infections. This can be as simple as getting a common cold, a stomach bug or fever, or something more serious, like Hashimoto's.

The importance of the immune system has gained more attention recently because of the covid-19 pandemic. For some this virus was like a mere cold; for others it was a death sentence. Still others survived but continue to have debilitating "long-hauler" symptoms months after being infected. The difference lies in the strength of the person's immune system. The coronavirus virus caused something called "cytokine storm," which modified the immune system, causing inflammation that led to damage of various parts of the body.

A similar situation happens in people with Hashimoto's, where an infection triggers their immune system to start destroying their thyroid and mitochondria. The good news is that there are ways you can retrain your immune system to stop damaging your thyroid gland and keep these chronic infections at bay.

Remember, Hashimoto's is caused by interactions between your genetic makeup and environmental factors. There is research that suggests a link between the disease and various kinds of infections.

The researchers found that there are several mechanisms through which these viruses trigger Hashimoto's. One of the most important things that viruses do when they attack our body is to highjack our immune system – they do this by modifying the immune cells. This leads to the creation of the antibodies that attack the thyroid and mitochondria, leading to Hashimoto's disease.

Another theory involves a mechanism called molecular mimicry. In this situation, certain pathogens can share similar molecular structures as the thyroid gland. When we get attacked by these pathogens, the body produces antibodies that not only hurt the pathogen, but the thyroid gland as well.

Viral infections like EBV (Epstein Barr Virus)

Viruses are the most common pathogen associated with Hashimoto's. In fact, thyroid disorders often start after a viral infection, particularly from Epstein Barr, the virus that causes mononucleosis. The worst part is that once you get infected by EBV, it stays in your body forever. It can lay in a dormant state for years, then can get reactivated in some individuals when their immunity is low. This reactivation of EBV can also lead to the development of Hashimoto's. In fact, a research study done in 2015 showed that a significant number of patients with Hashimoto's had a reactivation of EBV.

EBV infections lead to the development of Hashimoto's by modifying our immune system. We have two types of Immune cells – B cells and T cells. EBV virus infects both of them and alters their functioning, which leads to the development of anti-bodies that attack our body.

Also, EBV causes the destruction of mitochondria, which ultimately leads to all the thyroid symptoms we've discussed before. By destroying the mitochondria EBV not only decreases our immunity but also affects our body's ability to produce the necessary energy to sustain us.

Reactivation of EBV is very common, yet most people are unaware that it happened. Why? Because the symptoms are not as severe as the initial infection. Also, the test to check for acute EBV infection is not useful in this circumstance; more in-depth testing which we will talk about later, is required.

Parasites

Parasites are another form of pathogens that we get exposed to on a regular basis. Years ago, outbreaks of parasitic infections were a common occurrence; now, thanks to more effective safety measures and hygienic facilities, this doesn't happen so often, especially in developed countries. But we still get exposed to these parasites on regular basis.

You might be exposed to parasites while traveling, on camping or hiking trips, or eating in or taking out food from restaurants. Indeed, it is very easy to get exposed to these parasites, and when I check people for parasites the tests often come back positive.

Some of the parasites that have been linked to Hashimoto's disease are yersinia, giardia, entamoeba, and blastocystis.

Parasites cause immune dysfunction and lead to the activation of certain immune cells, inflammation, and, ultimately, trigger autoimmune conditions like Hashimoto's.

The most common symptoms associated with parasites are as follows:

1. Loss of appetite
2. Skin rash or hives
3. Histamine reactions
4. Allergies
5. Abdominal pain, bloating
6. Diarrhea or constipation
7. Upset stomach
8. Weight loss
9. Anemia
10. Weakness or fatigue
11. Anxiety or mood changes

A case report showed that a Hashimoto's patient was positive with Blastocystis Hominis. After he was treated for the Blastocystis the patient's antibodies and thyroid levels improved.

Additionally, a prospective cohort study looked for a connection between Blastocystis infection and Hashimoto's disease.

The patients were divided into three groups: the first had Hashimoto's disease but didn't have Blastocystis; the second had Hashimoto's and also had Blastocystis; and the third group was healthy. Researchers found that the second group had the highest level of thyroid antibodies and the lowest thyroid hormone levels. They were treated for the Blastocystis infection and saw significant improvement in their test results for TSH and TPO antibody levels.

The researchers found that Blastocystis causes immune dysfunction by increasing the levels of IL17, which is a kind of chemical mediator in your body that causes inflammation. Previous studies have shown that the higher the number of IL17, the lower the thyroid hormone levels. When the Blastocystis is treated, the IL17 decreases and that leads to improvement of Hashimoto's.

The problem with parasites is that they can be living in your system for several years without you even knowing about it. Many people associate parasites with symptoms like severe diarrhea or abdominal pain, but that might not be the case. The other issue is that the regular stool test will often miss the existence of these parasites. If your test comes back negative ask your physician to do a more detailed stool test.

Candida and Thyroid

Candida is a common fungus which lives in our body and normally does not affect our health. It is when there is an overgrowth of this fungus that it causes trouble.

Candida infections more commonly affect females, usually in the vaginal area and on the skin. More recently, we have identified another form of candida infection – intestinal candidiasis. This is when candida lives in your gut and overgrows there. Recent research also indicates that the overgrowth of candida is associated with several autoimmune diseases, especially Hashimoto's.

Why does candida overgrow in our body?

Our body is a place where several microorganisms live together happily. In our gut alone there are trillions of pathogens such as bacteria, fungus, and viruses cohabitating – balance is maintained by one pathogen keeping a check on the other. But sometimes this balance is disturbed and leads to overgrowth of one particular pathogen, like candida, which then starts hurting our body and can lead to the development of Hashimoto's.

What generally happens is that some of the good bacteria in our body is destroyed by processed food, antibiotics, stress, or through exposure to toxins. Once this good bacteria is compromised, there is nothing to fight the growth of candida. The overgrowth leads to inflammation and leaky gut, both of which are causes of Hashimoto's.

Below are the reasons for candida overgrowth:

1. Diets high in sugars, refined carbs
2. Medications like antibiotics
3. Reduced immunity through infections, or medications like steroids
4. Stress. Any kind of stress – be it physical, mental, or emotional – can cause candida overgrowth.
5. High alcohol intake

Symptoms of candida overgrowth:

1. Constipation, diarrhea, bloating, abdominal pain
2. Skin, vaginal and nail fungal infections
3. Feeling fatigued or tired
4. Sugar cravings
5. Brain fog and difficulty concentrating
6. Irritability, mood swings, depression, anxiety
7. Difficulty losing weight

How candida triggers Hashimoto's:

Candida has been associated with thyroid disorders, especially autoimmune thyroid disease. It has been seen that there is higher prevalence of candida infection in people with thyroid disease as compared to healthy people. There are various mechanisms through which candida affects our body and leads to development of Hashimoto's.

The first way is through molecular mimicry. As discussed earlier, this is when the molecular structure of a pathogen resembles that of our own tissues, which can trigger antibody production. One research study showed that candida antigens had immunological cross-reactivity with thyroid tissue, and that this can be the underlying mechanism by which candida triggers an autoimmune disease like Hashimoto's.

An overgrowth of candida in the gut also leads to inflammation, which destroys the intestinal protective lining. This leads to leaky gut, which, and previously discussed, is a trigger for Hashimoto's disease.

In addition, some people have genetic defects that prevent their body from fighting off candida. To clear candida infection we need healthy T cells, and those with compromised immunity cannot mount a proper response. This leads to the overgrowth of candida, inflammation, and, ultimately, the destruction of the mito-thyroid connection.

As you can see, candida infections can be a significant factor in triggering Hashimoto's and therefore must be part of the assessment process.

Lyme disease and other co-infections

Lyme disease is caused by a spirochaete called Borrelia burgdorferi and is mainly transmitted through tick bites. This infection often stays in the body and causes a host of problems, including Hashimoto's and other autoimmune diseases.

In the early stages of this infection, the spirochete grows in our system. But what we have found is that it can also hide in various body tissues, eventually altering our immune system and leading to Hashimoto's.

It has been postulated that chronic Lyme suppresses our immune system, this creating a pro-inflammatory state leading to Hashimoto's.

What we see is that the Borrelia is able to trick our immune system and survive in our body undetected and dormant for long periods of time. Then, when it sees an opportunity to get reactivated, it can simply modify our immune system and cause inflammation. Other co-infections include Babesia, Bartonella, Ehrlichia, and rickettsia – all of which are also associated with

Lyme disease. When searching for underlying causes of your Hashimoto's it's not enough to test for Lyme disease; you must also check for these co-infections as well.

It should be noted that while we don't have many research studies that link chronic Lyme infection with Hashimoto's, I have seen several patients improve after undergoing Lyme treatment.

CHAPTER 9

NUTRITIONAL DEFICIENCIES THAT TRIGGER HASHIMOTO'S

Our body (including the thyroid gland and mitochondria) needs many vitamins and minerals to function optimally. The only way we can get these nutrients into our body is through food or supplements, so making the right food choices is imperative, especially if we already have autoimmune disease.

That said, I have seen several people in my clinic who have tried to optimize their diet yet are still low in nutrients. Initially, I thought it was a lab error, but after I investigated I came to a shocking revelation: our food itself is deficient in these nutrients because our soil is deficient in these nutrients.

There was a research study done a while ago comparing the nutrient content in food in 1950 to that of 1999. What they found that food crops from 1999 were significantly lower in several nutrients like protein, calcium, phosphorus, iron, riboflavin (vitamin B2), and vitamin C. More recent studies show that our food now is low in several other nutrients like selenium, zinc, magnesium, potassium etc. In an effort to have better crop yields we have sacrificed their nutritional value.

Knowing this, I screen everyone with Hashimoto's for nutritional insufficiencies, and I often find they are low on several key nutrients needed for optimal thyroid and mitochondrial function.

Selenium

Selenium is an important micronutrient that has multiple functions in our body. Over the last several years its role has been studied in human physiology, and scientific reports have revealed its crucial role in the maintenance of immune-endocrine function, metabolism, and cellular homeostasis. In adults, the thyroid gland is the organ with the highest amount of selenium per gram of tissue.

Selenium in the form of selenoproteins is involved in the metabolism of thyroid hormones. These selenoproteins are part of two thyroid enzymes, deiodinases and glutathione peroxidase. These selenoproteins are also important for the proper functioning of mitochondria, and selenium deficiency is often associated with poor mitochondrial function.

These deiodinase enzymes are responsible for the conversion of T 4 hormone to T3 hormone. Inadequate levels of selenium can lead to impaired production of deiodinase, which in turn interferes with this conversion.

The other enzyme, glutathione peroxidase, is involved in antioxidant activities in the thyroid. During the production and conversion of thyroid hormones, free radicals are formed. If left alone these free radicals can damage your body, especially your mitochondria. Luckily the body has created defense mechanisms to get rid of these free radicals using glutathione peroxidase.

We can compare this to a factory that is manufacturing a finished product. During the process of making the product, waste material is generated. If not properly disposed of, this waste material will accumulate and become harmful for the factory and its workers. Similarly, if free radicals are not removed through detoxification, they accumulate and destroy your thyroid gland and mitochondria.

A study on 1,900 participants indicated an inverse relationship between serum selenium concentrations and thyroid volume, risk of goiter, and thyroid tissue damage in people with mild iodine deficiency.

Another study was conducted to see the role of selenium supplementation in people who have low thyroid and are already on levothyroxine. The results showed that the group with selenium supplementation had a reduction in thyroid antibodies, and saw improvement in their symptoms, while the group with just the levothyroxine did not.

Studies also show that selenium supplements help with improving mitochondrial function. Selenium not only protects the mitochondria from oxidative stress damage but also helps regenerate already damaged mitochondria.

Zinc

Zinc is an important mineral that supports immune function, as well as our skin, eyes, and heart health. It is also critical for our thyroid, as it regulates the deiodinases enzymes and plays a role in the conversion of T4 hormone to T3 hormone. People with a zinc deficiency can't convert T4 to T3, which is why levothyroxine doesn't help with their symptoms.

Studies have shown a direct correlation between zinc deficiency and low T3 levels; when these patients are supplemented with zinc, those levels improve. One study showed that zinc, when used alone or in conjunction with selenium, lowers TSH levels and increases the T3 and T4 levels.

Zinc is also critical for the proper functioning of mitochondria. A research study showed that low levels of zinc can interfere with mitochondrial energy production and metabolic activities. This means that zinc is essential for proper functioning of the mito-thyroid connection, and low levels can lead to the development of Hashimoto's disease.

Iodine

This is the most important mineral related to thyroid health. For those who already have thyroid issues it requires a delicate balancing act. We get iodine from our food, which is absorbed into the gut and then transported to the thyroid, where it is converted to thyroid hormone. An iodine deficiency, therefore, can lead to thyroid dysfunction.

There is also a debate about whether *too much* iodine can cause thyroid issues. Current research does indicate that too much iodine can lead to autoimmune thyroid disease like Hashimoto's. Moreover, excess iodine was shown to be dangerous to those who already have Hashimoto's disease. Why is this? Iodine temporarily shuts down the production of thyroid hormone. In most people, this was not a problem, as they were soon able to resume normal production, while those with Hashimoto's needed extra thyroid hormone medicine to keep their levels within the normal range.

Because of this, females with Hashimoto's have to be extra careful with iodine supplementation. I always recommend that Hashimoto's patients work with a Functional Medicine doctor who knows how their needs differ from other thyroid patients. Also, it is often possible to get enough iodine through food, so long as people consume the right foods on a regular basis.

The good news is that in most cases the negative effect of excess iodine lasted only a few weeks, and reducing the excess iodine was enough to get thyroid levels back to normal.

Iron

Iron is another mineral for thyroid health required for the production of thyroid hormones. It also helps with the conversion of T4 hormone to T3.

Iron deficiency is very common among middle-aged females, and it is estimated that 50-70% of women have low iron levels. Low iron levels lead to anemia and the common symptom of that is fatigue which is so common in Hashimoto's patients. Yet, surprisingly, I have found that most women with Hashimoto's have not gotten their iron levels checked.

Iron is also an important part of energy production because it regulates mitochondrial health. Iron deficiency leads to mitochondrial DNA damage as well as excess inflammation.

Bottom line, every Hashimoto's patient should get their levels checked to make sure low iron is not contributing to their illness.

B Vitamins

There are several B vitamins that are useful for thyroid and mitochondrial functioning, including Vitamin B2, B6, niacin, B9, and B12. People with Hashimoto's are deficient in at least one of these B vitamins, which affects their levels of thyroid production.

B vitamins are also involved in mitochondrial energy production, they destroy free radicals and thus prevent mitochondrial damage. On the other hand, low levels of these vitamins have been associated with poor mitochondrial function.

B12 is of particular concern for Hashimoto's patients. According to a one study, the prevalence of B12 deficiency in autoimmune thyroid patients was 28%; another determined it was even more common, with 55% found to be deficient in B12.

The reason for the high prevalence of B12 deficiency among Hashimoto's patients is pernicious anemia − an autoimmune disease that prevents people from absorbing B12 from food. People with Hashimoto's also have high rates of pernicious anemia. This is why it is very important to check for B12 deficiency in patients with Hashimoto's.

Vitamin D

Vitamin D is one of the most-widely studied vitamins. It has traditionally been associated with bone health, but in the last decade several studies have shown other benefits of vitamin D, one of which is the regulation of thyroid health, especially in Hashimoto's patients.

It has also been postulated that low vitamin D has been associated with the development of autoimmune diseases like Hashimoto's. Vitamin D is an important regulator of our immune system, and this regulation safeguards our body from getting autoimmune diseases.

When our body is deficient in vitamin D, our immune systems go crazy and start producing the antibodies that lead to Hashimoto's disease. Low vitamin D leads to the production of chemical mediators, which promotes inflammation in our body.

The interesting thing is that vitamin D deficiency is pervasive worldwide, affecting estimated one billion people or more, yet nobody is talking about it, or at least they're not doing anything to change the situation. I've seen several Hashimoto's patients whose vitamin D had never been checked, and supplementing with vitamin D makes a huge difference in their symptoms.

One of the major symptoms of low vitamin D is fatigue and brain fog issues, as well as higher inflammation and poor mitochondrial health, which again are symptoms of Hashimoto's.

The test for vitamin D is a simple one, available in every major lab, and should be standard for every Hashimoto's patient.

As you can, see there are several nutrients that are required for the proper functioning of the thyroid and mitochondria. And when they are low then it leads to the destruction of the mitothyroid connection which leads and exacerbates Hashimoto's symptoms.

PART III

> <

MY 3-STEP PROGRAM
TO REVERSE HASHIMOTO'S

I n the previous chapters we have explored the real reason people are suffering from Hashimoto's: the dysfunctional mito-thyroid connection. We also saw that there are various ways in which this connection can be broken, like consuming processed food; nutritional deficiencies; and exposure to toxins, stress, and infections. They trigger an autoimmune reaction which leads to the destruction of our mitochondria and thyroid.

The thyroid hormone levothyroxine, which is the conventional way of treating Hashimoto's, does not address this broken connection, which is why so many continue to suffer. Conventional medicine currently does not have any way to stop the autoimmune process, so the destruction of the thyroid and the rest of the body continues, leading to more symptoms.

Yet there is hope! My research has led me to create a simple 3- step process that helps you heal your Hashimoto's from inside out. This program focuses on first identifying the triggers that are responsible for your Hashimoto's. Then we work on addressing those triggers and on rejuvenating your mito-thyroid connection. The following chapters lay out these steps in a way that is easy to understand and you can start implementing them immediately.

CHAPTER 10

IDENTIFYING FOOD TRIGGERS

I introduced you to the concept of food sensitivity in Chapter 6. As mentioned, this is when your body starts reacting to certain foods you consume, eventually leading to Hashimoto's disease.

Most of the people I see with Hashimoto's have a food sensitivity to one or more food. There are certain foods that people are most commonly sensitive to, the reason being that they have been genetically modified in the last decade.

Again, the reason it's important to know about your food sensitivities is that they cause the destruction of mito-thyroid connection. Unless we remove these foods from your diet, your body will not heal.

The most common food that people are sensitive to are as follows:

1. Gluten
2. Dairy
3. Soy

4. Corn

5. Sugar

6. Processed red meat

Again, the reason most people are sensitive to these foods is that they have been genetically modified. Even the dairy industry has been known to keep their livestock in inhumane conditions, and when we consume the dairy products from this livestock our body just rejects them. Sugar is another inflammatory product that is present almost in any food you buy off the self. Added sugar in our diet has increased considerably in the last decade and it has led to an increased incidence of Hashimoto's disease.

Below is a questionnaire you can use to help figure out if you have food sensitivities.

1. Do you have nausea or vomiting?

2. Do you suffer from constipation or diarrhea?

3. Do you suffer from heartburn or acid reflux?

4. Do you suffer from bloating?

5. Are you excessively full after meals?

6. Do you suffer from stomach pains or cramps?

7. Do you have reactions to several foods?

8. Do you feel tired after eating?

9. Do you feel irritable or anxious?

10. Do you have to clear your throat often?

11. Do you suffer from a runny nose, or sneezing?

12. Do have itchy skin or hives?

If you answered yes to any of these questions, you might have issues with food sensitivities. Go to Reversinghashimotobook. com for a more comprehensive quiz that will give you an idea about how serious your food sensitivity is.

Let's say this questionnaire tells you that you might have food sensitivities — how do you find out exactly which food(s) are affecting you?

The good news is that there are now several tests available that can help you identify food sensitivities.

1. Food allergy test: As we discussed earlier, food allergies are different from food sensitivities and often have clearer symptoms. However, if you are unsure about what foods you are allergic to, these tests are helpful. They check for IgE antibodies, which are secreted as soon as your body gets in contact with food that your body is allergic to. By measuring the levels of these IgE antibodies in your blood, we learn the severity of the food allergy.

2. Food sensitivity test: This kind of test checks for IgG antibodies in your system. IgG antibodies are different then IgE antibodies in that they don't show symptoms immediately. IgG antibodies generally cause more delayed symptoms in the body, making it difficult to know which food caused the reaction. These tests are therefore useful in identifying the culprit(s).

Please note that just because you have IgG antibodies to a certain food doesn't mean it is causing harm to your body. Therefore, the results of this test need to be interpreted by a Functional Medicine expert who has experience with food sensitivities and can help create the right food plan for you.

CHAPTER 11

IDENTIFYING TOXIN TRIGGERS

Previously we discussed the numerous toxins in our environment and how it is almost impossible to avoid exposure. Remember, while our body has natural mechanisms in place to get rid of toxins, overloading it with these substances leads to diseases like Hashimoto's.

Reducing our toxic burden makes it possible for our body to handle the toxins on its own. That said, we may need some extra support to do so.

Before we get into that, let's talk first about how you can figure out if you are toxic. Answering the following questions is a good start.

1. Are you sensitive to strong smells around you?
2. Do you have numbness, tingling, or itching in the hands and feet?
3. Do you have reactions to various kinds of food?
4. Do you feel fatigued or tired?

5. Do you suffer from mood changes, irritability, depression, or anxiety?

6. Do you have an inability to concentrate and multitask?

7. Did your current or any previous house ever have any water leaks or water damage?

8. Did your current or any previous house ever have a musty odor in the basement?

9. Do you have skin issues (i.e., eczema, rash, hives, and itching)?

10. Have you ever seen mold in your house?

11. Do you have metal or amalgam fillings in your teeth?

12. Do you get exposed to harsh chemicals (cleaning agents, glue, gas, et cetera)?

13. Does your drinking water come from a private well or a city water supply?

14. Are pesticides or herbicides (i.e., bug or weed killers; flea and tick sprays; collars; powders; or shampoos) used in your home, garden, or surrounding areas?

If you answered yes to any of these questions there's a chance that toxins are playing a role in your Hashimoto's.

I have developed a score that gives you a better idea about the toxic load in your body; for that, go to reversinghashimotobook. com and take the quiz.

The above questionnaire is a good screening tool, but to know for sure if toxins are playing a role in your Hashimoto's you need to do toxin testing. Unfortunately, we don't have one single test that checks for these toxins; you have to test for them one at a time.

The other issue is that regular labs don't offer testing for these toxins, so you need to work with a Functional Medicine provider to get them done.

As toxins are present in different parts of our body, different testing methods have been devised for them.

1. **Heavy metals:** Recall that there are several heavy metals like mercury, lead, and arsenic that can lead to Hashimoto's. All of these needs to be checked to see if they are present in your body and at what levels.

   There are various tests used to check the presence of these heavy metals in your body. The most common is a blood test, however, this doesn't give the total amount of heavy metals in your body, nor does it test for the various types of heavy metals. Another method is hair analysis, which is good for some metals like mercury but might not be the best for others like arsenic. Urine levels are more stable and give us a better evaluation of chronic exposure to heavy metals. It also can be done with a home kit. For these reasons, urine is my preferred method to check for these heavy metals.

2. **Environmental toxins:** There is currently no standard lab that offers tests for environmental toxins. The good news is that there are certain specialized labs that do offer them. As we have thousands of toxins in our environment, there is no way to check for all of them. But we can check the most important ones

like organophosphate pesticides, phthalates, benzene, xylene, vinyl chloride, pyrethroid insecticides, acrylamide, perchlorate, diphenyl phosphate, ethylene oxide, and acrylonitrile. You can talk to your Functional Medicine doctor to learn more about this test and how to get it done.

3. **Mold toxins:** Again, there is no standard blood test to check for all the different kinds of mold toxins that can lead to Hashimoto's disease. However, there are urine tests available to check for mycotoxins, which have been linked to various chronic diseases. These tests tell you exactly what kind of mold toxins are in your body. Once you know that you can work with your Functional Medicine doctor to get rid of them.

The questionnaire can be a very helpful tool to give you an idea of whether your body is harboring too many toxins. However, you will need some of these advanced tests in order to check for the specific culprits.

CHAPTER 12

IDENTIFYING STRESS TRIGGERS

As we learned earlier, stress can be a major factor in your Hashimoto's, though it is one overlooked by many people. Time and time again, I have seen people who were diagnosed with Hashimoto's after dealing with a high-stress situation such as a difficult relationship, work stress, pregnancy, financial stress, et cetera.

Patients often say to me, "Everyone has stress, so why do only a few develop Hashimoto's?" The answer is that we all have a different genetic make-up and yours might make you more susceptible to Hashimoto's. Another reason could be the way your body processes stress. Research now shows that how we *perceive* our stress is just as determinative of the outcome as the stress itself, if not more so.

Below is a great perceived stress response questionnaire used by several psychological institutes. It can help you identify whether your body is more susceptible to the effects of stress.

0 = Never 1 = Almost Never 2 = Sometimes 3 = Fairly Often
= Very Often*

1. In the last month, how often have you been upset because of something that happened unexpectedly?
2. In the last month, how often have you felt you were unable to control the important things in your life?
3. In the last month, how often have you felt nervous and "stressed"?
4. In the last month, how often have you felt confident about your ability to handle your personal problems?
5. In the last month, how often have you felt that things were going your way?
6. In the last month, how often have you found that you could not cope with all the things that you had to do?
7. In the last month, how often have you been able to control irritations in your life?
8. In the last month, how often have you felt that you were on top of things?
9. In the last month, how often have you been angered because of things that were outside of your control?
10. In the last month, how often have you felt difficulties were piling up so high that you could not overcome them?

A score of more than 12 can signify that your body is more susceptible to stress.

* "The Perceived Stress Scale (PSS) developed by **Cohen, Kamarck and Mermelstein**"

After taking the questionnaire you might be able to identify whether you have stress-related issues. You might also be wondering whether there is any testing available to check the level of stress in your body. The answer is yes.

Remember how we spoke about the hormone cortisol, and how chronic high levels of it lead to all the harmful effects of stress? Well, we have ways to check these cortisol levels.

The interesting thing about cortisol is that its levels fluctuate throughout the day. In the morning when you wake up the cortisol levels are high, during the day they fluctuate based on what activities you are doing, and at night they are at their lowest so you can easily go to sleep.

This means that checking cortisol levels only once will not accurately determine if you have a problem. We need to check cortisol levels multiple times a day, and while we can do this through the blood there is an easier way. It has been shown that saliva tests for cortisol levels are just as accurate as blood levels, and it's certainly more pleasant than being stuck with a needle over and over again.

I regularly order cortisol levels for my patients and they often come back abnormal, so it is important to check them to help identify if stress is playing a role in your Hashimoto's.

CHAPTER 13

IDENTIFYING HASHIMOTO-TRIGGERING INFECTIONS

We saw previously that infections – such as viruses, bacteria, parasites, and Lyme disease – can be a root cause of Hashimoto's disease. It can be difficult to identify these pathogens as the cause because they often lie dormant in our body for several years. When they reactivate, they trigger the immune system, which leads to the development of antibodies and eventually the destruction of our mito-thyroid connection.

We are again going to use a questionnaire as a screening tool to determine whether underlying infections might be the reason for your Hashimoto's. It was challenging to narrow down the right questions because there are so many different kinds of infections that can lead to Hashimoto's, but I've found these to be a good starting point.

1. Have you ever had a tick bite?
2. Have you ever been diagnosed with EBV or mononucleosis?

3. Do you take long time to recover from illness of any kind?

4. Do you get frequent colds/sinus infections or bronchitis?

5. Do you have joint pain or swelling?

6. Do you have muscle pains or stiffness?

7. Do you feel tired or fatigued?

8. Do you have fever or chills?

9. Do you have tingling, numbness, burning or stabbing sensations?

10. Do you have problems with sleep?

11. Do you have forgetfulness, or feel your memory is not that great as before?

12. Do you have frequent mood swings, irritability or depression?

The above questionnaire can help you determine whether infections might be playing role in your health. You can take the online quiz to know your score at Reversinghashimoto-book.com. Now, sometimes even people with low scores have underlying infections, so it's important to talk to your health professional about your symptoms to decide whether further testing is a good idea.

EBV (Ebstein Barr Virus) Testing

EBV is very common worldwide and most of the time it's a latent infection so people don't even know they have it. Once you get EBV, the virus stays in your body and never leaves. Furthermore, even in the latent stages this virus has been linked to various kinds of autoimmune infections and cancers.

A blood test can determine if you have EBV; the problem is that most of the time the test ordered is the Monospot test, which does not show the complete breakdown of all the antibodies, so we don't know if the EBV has reactivated. The tests that you need are:

1. Anti- VCA IgM and IgG

2. Anti-EA IgG

3. Antibody to Nuclear Antigen (EBNA)

The interpretation of these tests is complicated and should be done by a medical provider who understands the results.

Testing for Parasites

Checking for parasites can be very tricky because oftentimes they hide in our body.

Most of the parasites I have mentioned before remain in your gut so that's the best possible place to check for them. A stool test makes the most sense; the problem is the old method involves examining it under a microscope. Even then, the parasites are difficult to see, and/or the stool sample might not have enough parasites in it.

Using a combination of methods increases the probability of finding these parasites. For example, some lab companies are offering an advanced stool analysis where they combine the microscopic method with enzyme immunoassay and Polymerase chain reaction. These are the tests you need to ask your Functional Medicine practitioner to order to get a clear answer.

Testing for Candida Infection

There are different kinds of testing available to check for the overgrowth of candida in the gut.

1. Blood test

This is the simplest way to check for candida. Your body produces antibodies against candida and you can measure these antibodies in your blood. That said, it is also the most difficult test to interpret.

The typical candida antibodies are IgG, IgM, and candida complex. The results of this test need to be interpreted carefully, as sometimes it can show past infection but not a current one. The other problem is that this test might show that you don't have current antibodies again candida when in reality your body is so immunocompromised that it is *not able* to produce these antibodies.

2. Stool test

Advanced Functional Medicine stool tests can be used to identify candida in your gut. This is similar to the stool test we discussed above to check for parasites. They try to culture yeast in the gut and give you the extent of overgrowth. The problem with these tests is that candida is very difficult to grow outside the body, therefore, it sometimes yields a false negative.

3. Organic acid testing

There are certain Functional Medicine tests that check for organic acids in the urine, which are metabolites produced by candida. Tartaric acid and arabinose are the most common organic acids, which are associated with candida overgrowth.

As you can see, the testing for candida is complicated and requires careful interpretation by an experienced Functional Medicine physician to determine if you have candida overgrowth.

Testing for Chronic Lyme and Co-infections

Testing chronic Lyme infection is very challenging at this point in time. Regular labs do offer tests that provide some insight, but they might not be doing an in-depth analysis.

There are other labs, however, that offer a more detailed analysis of Lyme disease, such as Western blot testing. They can also be very helpful in diagnosing co-infections like Bartonella, babesia, and ehrlichiosis.

CHAPTER 14

IDENTIFYING NUTRITIONAL DEFICIENCY TRIGGERS

We saw before how the mito-thyroid connection gets broken because of low levels of certain vitamins and minerals. In fact, most people with Hashimoto's are low in one or more vitamins or minerals. This can be the case even if your diet is very healthy.

There are several signs and symptoms that can help you determine whether you might have any nutritional insufficiencies. I have developed this questionnaire that might give you some insight.

1. Do you feel exhausted or sore after exercise?

2. Do you feel sleepy or sluggish?

3. Do you have trouble with concentration or focus?

4. Do you have pain all over your body or suffer from migraines?

5. Do you have mood change issues like depression/ anxiety?

6. Do you feel dizzy?

7. Do you have weight issues – specifically, are you unable to lose weight?

8. Do have feel a burning or tingling sensation?

9. Do you have issues with brittle nails?

10. Do you have hair loss or hair thinning?

11. Do you suffer from dry skin?

If you answer yes to any of these questions you may have nutritional deficiencies. You can take online quiz by going to reversinghashimotobook.com and get your score for nutritional deficiencies.

Advanced Testing for the Nutritional Deficiencies

There are so many nutrients needed for thyroid and mito-chondrial function that to check each one separately would be difficult, to say the least. Fortunately, there are now several specialized labs that can get information about all these nutrients with just one sample.

That said, while some of these nutrients like vitamin D, magnesium and iron can easily be checked through regular labs, to get accurate levels for others we need advanced Functional Medicine labs.

A note about checking Vitamin B12: the blood test usually ordered to check these levels may not be sufficient. To make sure a B12 deficiency does not go undetected, I suggest looking at different markers like MMA (Methylmalonic acid) and homocysteine levels in conjunction with blood levels of vitamin B12.

Iodine testing: There are different ways of testing iodine, and each has its own advantages. Most common is checking iodine in the blood, followed by a urine iodine test and an iodine urine loading test. Out of the three, the urine iodine test is the simplest as it can be done at home. Studies also show that it is very reliable.

Iron levels: Many doctors only order iron levels; however, I don't believe this is sufficient. To get a complete picture of iron levels in the body I recommend ordering iron levels with CBC (Complete Blood Count) and ferritin levels.

CHAPTER 15

THE MITO-THYROID DIET

Throughout this book we have been talking about all the factors, external and internal, that destroy the mito-thyroid connection and cause Hashimoto's. Now we'll move on to ways in which we can start fixing this connection and feel better.

One of the cornerstones of this program is the Mito-Thyroid Diet. As I said previously, food is medicine but it can also be your enemy. Surprisingly, while there are several diets on the market for various diseases, there are no specific diets for Hashimoto's; this, despite the fact that we know these patients have their own nutritional needs in order to restore proper functioning of the thyroid and mitochondria.

Food is one of the best ways to get those nutrients. After years of treating Hashimoto's patients and researching the disease, I have developed a diet that not only reduces inflammation in your body but also helps rejuvenate your thyroid and mitochondria.

The Mito-Thyroid Diet focuses on incorporating good fats and high-quality protein, as that helps the mito-thyroid connection. It has a low glycemic index, and is gluten-free, which helps with reducing inflammation in your body. It also includes tons of non-starchy vegetables, as they have high amounts of antioxidants and nutrients that are needed by your body.

It is important to understand the rationale of this diet so that you can incorporate it into your life.

The Mito-Thyroid Diet is founded on the following principles:

1. First Principle: remove foods that are causing damage to the mito-thyroid connection. As mentioned, this includes sugary foods, processed foods, trans-fats, gluten, dairy, soy, and corn.

2. Second principle: Add foods that repair the mito-thyroid connection. These include things like good fats, high-quality proteins, nuts and seeds.

3. Third Principle: Add antioxidant-rich foods that reduce inflammation and stop the destruction of the mito-thyroid connection, such as green leafy vegetables, some fruits, and gluten-free grains.

First principle: Removing foods that are damaging the mito-thyroid connection

In Chapter 6, we covered foods that are harmful to the mito-thyroid connection. Most people with Hashimoto's disease have a sensitivity to these foods and are advised to avoid them. I have personally seen numerous Hashimoto's patients get better after they remove the following toxic foods from their diet.

1. Gluten
2. Dairy
3. Soy
4. Corn
5. Sugar
6. Processed red meat
7. Other processed foods

It's important to note that you will need to eliminate these foods for at least four weeks. The reason for this is that once you consume any food you are sensitive to, your body produces antibodies that can stay in your system for three to four weeks. Most people will eliminate these foods for one week, get discouraged when they don't see a change, and go back to eating them. I urge you not to give up, because with perseverance improvement is right around the corner.

Another common mistake people make is that they don't eliminate these foods completely from their diet; instead, they merely eat them less often. What they don't realize is that their body is still making those harmful antibodies.

Some people will ask if they can cut out these foods one at a time, but at that rate it can take you four to five months to find the culprit. I recommend trying to eliminate all of them at once, as this will speed up your progress and get you feeling better faster.

Second principle: Adding foods that fix the mito-thyroid connection

These foods include:

1. **Good Fats:**

   Fats are very important for the proper functioning of mitochondria and thyroid. They are fuel for your body and are needed for the absorption of certain vitamins and minerals. That said, not all fats are created equal – there are good fats and there are bad fats. Good fats like Omega-3 help us naturally get rid of inflammation. They are also used to make cell membranes, especially nerve cells. In fact, nearly 60% of your brain is fat.

   Bad fats are generally trans-fats that are present in fried food or fast food. They have been associated with heart disease, strokes, and inflammation in the body. Though in USA the sale of trans-fats has been banned, the food industry has found innovative ways to include them in your diet, so always be sure to the read labels.

   The difference between these fats is their underlying chemical structure. The structure of all fats includes a chain of carbon atoms that are bonded with hydrogen atoms. What varies is the chain, the length of carbon, or the number of hydrogen bonds. These minor changes in their chemical structure equals significant changes to their properties.

Below are the foods which might have trans-fats and therefore should be completely removed from your diet:

1. Fried foods like French fries, donuts, and most battered food
2. Microwave popcorn
3. Margarine
4. Some baked food like cakes, cookies, and pies

Other bad fats include certain kinds of vegetable oils like canola oil, soybean oil, peanut oil, safflower oil, and sunflower oil, all of which increase inflammation in our body. The reason is that they are very high in Omega-6 fatty acids. In low quantity Omega-6 is fine, but high consumption is a problem, especially for Hashimoto's patients. Unfortunately, the standard American diet is very high in Omega-6 and very low in Omega-3.

Now let's talk about the good fats you need to reduce inflammation and help heal your mito-thyroid connection.

These fats can be divided into various categories, such as:

1. Saturated fats – coconut oil, ghee. For a long time, these fats were labeled dangerous so many people avoided them completely. But new research suggests that they are actually good for your heart and can also help improve your cholesterol. That said, it is important to source them from a reputable place and they should not be processed.

2. Monosaturated fats – olive oil, avocados, nuts (i.e., almonds, pecans). A research study from the 1960s

revealed that people living in Mediterranean region had a low rate of heart disease. The reason for this, they figured out, was the high consumption of monosaturated fat (olive oil).

The majority of the fats in avocados are in the form of monounsaturated fatty acid – or oleic acid – which is helpful in regulating your cholesterol and can actually be helpful in reducing bad cholesterol. Avocados are also full of nutrients, including vitamin K, folate, vitamin C, potassium, vitamin B5, vitamin B6, and vitamin E. Avocados actually have more potassium than bananas, and their high fiber content make them helpful in treating gut dysfunction and detoxification through regular bowel movements. Also, the soluble fiber in avocados acts as prebiotics and helps to improve your gut microbiome.

3. Polyunsaturated fats – fatty fishes, walnuts, flaxseeds, and chia seeds. This is the form of fat that will help you the most. For example, Omega-3 fats are healing to the thyroid and help reduce inflammation as well.

Fatty fish like mackerel, anchovy, sardines, salmon, and herring should be included in your diet on a daily basis if possible. They are not only good sources of Omega-3 fatty acids like DHA and EPA, they are also low in carbs and high in good quality proteins.

A study was done to assess the effect of certain kinds of fish on the thyroid. Participants were divided into two groups – one that ate swordfish or oily fish high in Omega-3, and the other that ate different kinds of fish. Researchers found the level of thyroid antibodies was significantly lower in the group that consumed the fish high in Omega-3.

You do have to be cautious about the source of your fish, as these days most of our fish is high in mercury. Be sure the fish you eat is wild caught.

2. **Nuts and Seeds**

These foods are extremely important and yet are often ignored by a lot of people. Nuts (i.e., Brazil nuts, almonds, walnuts, pine nuts, and pecans) and seeds (i.e., pumpkin seeds and sunflower seeds) are packed with powerful nutrients and are very helpful for people with Hashimoto's. They are good sources of various nutrients like selenium, Omega-3, and other things that help to heal the thyroid and mitochondria.

Chia seeds and flax seeds are especially good sources of Omega-3 fatty acids, especially for vegetarians or people who don't want to eat fish. They are also low in calories, and high in protein and fiber. Chia and flax are rich in ALA (alpha-linolenic acid), which needs to be converted to EPA and DHA. It should be noted, however, that some people have genetic variations that interfere with this conversion.

Similarly, sunflower seeds, pumpkin seeds are also very healthy and can help to reduce inflammation in your body.

Nuts like almonds, walnuts, and pecans contain a lot of good fats that help to heal your mito-thyroid connection. They are also good sources of protein, fiber, and also other vitamins too.

Brazil nuts in particularly are a very good source of selenium. Recall that selenium is an important mineral needed for the proper functioning of the thyroid; unfortunately, most people with Hashimoto's are low in selenium. One single Brazil nut contains 68 to 91 micrograms; most people with thyroid dysfunction need anywhere from 100 to 200 mcg of selenium. This means you only need to eat 1 to 2 Brazil nuts a day to fulfill your selenium requirement and keep your thyroid in good shape.

A concern many people have about nuts and seeds is that they are high in phytic acid levels, which can interfere with the absorption of minerals or cause sensitivities. But if you soak these nuts and seeds and sprout them, it reduces the level of phytic acid dramatically.

3. **Oysters and Other Seafood**

Oysters are one of the foods with the highest zinc content. Remember, zinc is another essential mineral needed for the thyroid to function properly, and zinc deficiency is a major cause of low thyroid. Zinc controls thyroid hormone production by regulating deiodinases enzymes. Zinc is also involved in the conversion of T4 hormone to T3 hormone. Other seafood like a cooked lobster and king crab also has a good amount of zinc in them. Seafood is also low in calories and packed with nutrients.

4. **Good Quality Protein:**

Proteins are the building blocks of our body and we all know how important they are for proper health, including the thyroid. In Hashimoto's patients, protein is especially critical as it reduces inflammation and helps modulate our immune system. These proteins also help to reduce weight by controlling the insulin surges that typically happen with carbs. Good quality protein is also high in antioxidants and thus safeguards your mito-thyroid connection.

It's important to understand that not all proteins are created equal. Poor quality proteins promote inflammation in your body, and they are difficult to digest. This means instead of helping your body they actually damage your thyroid gland.

One of the most common examples of bad protein are whey protein supplements. The whey protein is derived from dairy and leads to increased inflammatory markers in Hashimoto's patients. Also concerning are processed meats, which are very high in artificial additives and significantly increase the inflammation markers. The industrialized poultry and meat industry is a major reason for the increased the number of people with Hashimoto's disease. This livestock is treated with artificial hormones, and their feed is very low in nutrients. It is also very high in gluten and grains, which leads to inflammation. When we consume these types of poultry and meats, it causes inflammation in our bodies and leads to Hashimoto's disease.

Some of the sources of good quality proteins are:

1. Wild-caught fish like mackerel, anchovy, sardines, salmon, and herring
2. Grass-fed beef

3. Organic, pasture-raised chicken

4. Nuts and seeds like almonds, chia and flax seeds

   Of the best ways to get protein in your diet is through smoothies. I like my morning smoothie and I rotate my protein powders (there are a variety of these powders so make sure you look at the ingredients carefully). Starting your day strong with a good protein smoothie will go a long way in reducing inflammation, promoting weight loss, and keeping your energy level up.

Third principle: reducing inflammation through foods high in antioxidants

1. **Colorful vegetables**

   Non-starchy vegetables are the cornerstone of this diet plan. We need to include as many colorful vegetables as we can. Each of these colors has its own benefit for the mito-thyroid connection. Non-starchy vegetables are also low-carb and anti-inflammatory. Most starchy vegetables, on the other hand, have a lot of carbohydrates and can also increase your insulin levels.

   Starchy vegetables that you should avoid are:

1. Potatoes

2. Sweet potatoes/yams

3. Plantain

4. Pumpkin

5. Squash

6. Corn

People are always asking me why we should avoid some of these vegetables, such as sweet potatoes, which are thought to be healthy. While sweet potatoes are better than regular potatoes, they still have a lot of carbohydrates and will not let your thyroid heal properly. This means you need to avoid them, at least until your mito-thyroid connection has healed.

Now let's talk about the vegetables that you need to include in your diet. Greens are a very important part of this food plan and should be consumed on a daily basis. Green leafy vegetables like spinach, kale, chard, and collard and mustard greens contain many nutrients, such as vitamins B and C and iron, that heal the mito-thyroid connection. They are also high in antioxidants which help with decreasing inflammation and thus safeguard the mito-thyroid connection. Kale is especially high in an antioxidant compound called quercetin, which has been shown to reduce inflammation in the body. Similarly, spinach is high in vitamin C, beta carotene, and other antioxidants which help your mito-thyroid connection.

Other vegetables that are very helpful for restoring this connection are those containing sulfur, such as broccoli, Brussel sprouts, cabbage, cauliflower, and asparagus.

These vegetables have high levels of sulforaphane, powerful antioxidants, and detoxifiers, all of which reduce inflammation and protect the thyroid and mitochondria from oxidative damage.

Traditional thinking held that these foods are goitrogens, which means they can actually harm your thyroid. This was based on a study in 1928, where scientists saw that rabbits eating lots of cabbage have thyroid issues. The reason was that these goitrogens can interfere with the proper absorption of iodine in the thyroid. But we have not seen any good research study in humans since that time that proves that goitrogens should be completely avoided. In fact, most studies indicate that these cruciferous vegetables can be beneficial to the thyroid, especially for people with Hashimoto's, as they reduce underlying inflammation.

Seaweeds deserve special mention here, as they are a very good source of iodine which again is an essential nutrient for thyroid functioning. Nori, kelp, and wakame all have good amounts of iodine and can be helpful.

Seaweed also has other nutrients with potent antioxidant powers and can help protect your thyroid from inflammation. It is an excellent source of fiber that keeps your gut is in good shape and can help with constipation, which several thyroid patients suffer from.

All other non-starchy vegetables are also beneficial for your thyroid and should be consumed daily. I call these "free" foods, meaning you can have them as much as you like without worrying about any issues. In fact I suggest to all my Hashimoto's patients that more than half of their dinner/lunch plate should be vegetables. That's how important they are for healing the thyroid gland.

2. **Fruits**

Fruits are an important part of our diet, and most of us like to consume them on regular basis. When it comes to healing the thyroid, however, we need to choose fruits that are high in antioxidants and also low in carbohydrates. We also have to be careful about eating fruits because they contain sugar.

Yes, these are natural sugars, but they can still be harmful to your mito-thyroid connection. Therefore as we are trying to heal this connection it is very important to restrict the number of fruits we eat to one serving a day.

Let's look at some of the fruits you should include with this diet.

Blueberries:
Blueberries are one of the best fruits to support your thyroid gland and should be a part of your daily diet. They are a super-food meaning they have a low glycemic index, are very low in carbohydrates, and are high in vitamin C, vitamin K, and manganese – all of which are required to support your thyroid gland.

Blueberries are high in several antioxidant compounds, especially flavonoids. In fact, out of all the fruits blueberries have the highest amount of these antioxidant compounds. These flavonoids not only reduce inflammation in your body but also help in reducing reactive oxygen species which are responsible for thyroid gland damage. The best part is that blueberries don't lose their health benefits when they are frozen, so you can stock them for year-round use.

Strawberries
Strawberries are another fruit that are both delicious and loaded with many nutrients that are beneficial for the thyroid. They are also relatively low in natural sugar as compared to other fruits, and are a good source of vitamin C – around 51 mg per serving. This might seem like a small amount, but getting it on a daily basis can be very helpful. Also, strawberries have a significant amount of phytonutrients like anthocyanins, ellagic acid and ellagitannins that help with reducing inflammation in your thyroid gland. These also help with optimizing your body's natural detox system.

Strawberries can be a good addition to your morning smoothies, along with or in place of blueberries.

Pomegranate
Pomegranate is a less popular super fruit that has several health benefits, most of which come from polyphenol compounds. These polyphenols are what give this fruit its color.

They also help remove free radicals from the body, which in turn decreases inflammation and protects your thyroid gland.

Pomegranates are also rich in antioxidants; in fact, pomegranate juice has three times the antioxidants as wine and green tea.

This also protects your brain and can be helpful for brain fog, as well as pain. Chronic pain is another most common symptom of thyroid disorder.

Another issue with thyroid patients is high cholesterol. Most of the time thyroid disorder causes high levels of LDL cholesterol (aka "bad" cholesterol), which can lead to future cardiac problems. Pomegranate juice has been shown to lower LDL levels.

Pomegranate has a very distinct taste so it might take time for you to adjust to it. The easiest way to consume this fruit is by drinking the juice, but make sure you don't drink more than a small shot of it as it does contain sugar.

Apples
Apples are one of the most popular fruits worldwide. They also have several health benefits, as they contain several vitamins and minerals, including phytonutrients. The majority of these phytonutrients are in the skin so make sure to eat that.

One of the most important phytonutrients is quercetin, which reduces inflammation and is helpful for people with mast cell disorder or allergies. Quercetin, along with other phytochemicals like catechins, chlorogenic acid, is a powerful antioxidant and protects your thyroid gland from free radical damage. Apples also contain a soluble fiber called pectin, which promotes gut health.

3. Gluten-free Grains

Gluten-free grains are also an important part of the mito-thyroid diet. They have several health benefits but, like fruits, we have to be careful with the serving size. I recommend one-half cup of cooked grains per day. These gluten-free grains use various mechanisms to help with reducing inflammation in your body and thus protect your mito-thyroid connection.

Gluten-free grains allowed on this diet are:

- Quinoa
- Amaranth
- Arrowroot
- Buckwheat
- Millet
- Brown rice, including wild rice
- Sorghum
- Teff
- Gluten-free oats

One of the main benefits of these gluten free grains is that they have several vitamins and minerals like iron, magnesium, vitamin B2, manganese, and zinc. All these vitamins and minerals support thyroid gland health, directly or indirectly.

Another benefit of these grains, especially quinoa, is that they are high in antioxidant compounds like quercetin and kaempferol. And we already know that quercetin is very effective in reducing inflammation and safeguarding your mito-thyroid connection.

Most of these gluten-free grains also have a low glycemic index. Glycemic index is used to measure the amount of sugar spikes a particular food causes − the lower the glycemic index, the less the food raises sugar levels in your blood. Rice is among gluten-free grains we have to be careful with, especially white rice, which can raise your sugar levels. Brown rice is a better choice, as is quinoa. Also, quinoa has one of the lowest glycemic indexes − just 53.

Most of these gluten-free grains are also high in fiber, which prevents insulin spikes that occur when you consume carbohydrates. Insulin in excess causes inflammation, which is the root of thyroid disorder. Also, the high fiber keeps your gut in healthy shape by directly influencing the growth of good bacteria there. Remember, there is a strong correlation between the gut and the thyroid gland. Poor gut health increases inflammation in your body and thus hurts the mito-thyroid connection. So you see, these gluten-free grains are a key piece of the plan to improve thyroid health.

CHAPTER 16

WENDY'S EASY WEIGHT LOSS STORY

Do you remember Wendy, the thirty-two-year-old who was suffering from thyroid issues and had gained fifty pounds she was unable to lose? She was having body image issues and fearing she would look ugly for the rest of her life. She tried restricting her calories, even to the point of passing out a couple of times.

When she saw me in the clinic we spoke in detail about the mito-thyroid connection. We dug deeper to find the root cause of her problem and identified food sensitivities to gluten, dairy, soy, corn, and some other foods. Because of this food sensitivity problem, she had developed a leaky gut and that led to the development of Hashimoto's. These food sensitivities had also destroyed her mito-thyroid connection, which had led to weight gain. During her five-year struggle with Hashimoto's, she never imagined that food sensitivities could be the culprit.

Wendy was so desperate to lose weight that she had focused on the quantity of food – eating as few calories as possible – when she should have been focusing on the quality. So this is what we worked on. We made a plan that removed all the foods her body was sensitive to and introduced foods that helped her to restore the mito-thyroid connection. It took some convincing to get her to try the green smoothie, but now she loves it so much she has one every morning for breakfast. Within six weeks of starting this food plan, Wendy started losing weight – around fifteen pounds. We added some supplements to help with her leaky gut and to support her mito-thyroid connection, and within three months she had lost forty-five pounds.

Wendy couldn't believe that it happened just by making some changes to her diet. As with anybody who has struggled with weight, she dreaded diets that required her to starve herself. While on our diet she had so much to eat that she always felt full and her craving for sweet food went away.

Like most people carrying extra weight, those with Hashimoto's tend to focus on calories. When we shift this focus to the quality of food, the weight comes off easily.

CHAPTER 17

SUPPLEMENTS SUPPORTING THYROID AND MITOCHONDRIA

N ow we turn to the supplements you can use to support your mito-thyroid connection. There are several supplements that are good for both thyroid and mitochondria, but here I am going to talk about the absolute musts for Hashimoto's patients.

Selenium: We have seen previously that selenium is an important mineral for thyroid hormone production and mitochondrial health.

A study was conducted to find the right dosage of selenium. Participants were given either 100 ug/ day or 200 ug/day for nine months and their levels of thyroid antibodies were monitored. The results showed that the group who were given 200 ug/day showed a significant reduction in thyroid antibodies while the group getting 100 ug/day did not; therefore, they concluded that the proper selenium dosage is at least 200 ug/day. I feel the right dosage of selenium should be between 150 and 200 mcg/

daily, depending upon whether you are eating selenium-rich foods or not. There are different forms of selenium supplements in the market, but not all of them are good for your thyroid. The best form for absorption is selenomethionine, so make sure your supplement contains this ingredient. A dose of more than 200ug should not be taken for long periods as there is a potential risk of toxicity, but most people do fine if they stick with the recommended dosage.

Zinc: As we have seen previously, zinc is needed for the production of thyroid hormones, as well as for the conversion of T4 hormone to T3. There are some dietary sources of zinc, but the problem is that the zinc is poorly absorbed from food. To bypass these issues the newer zinc supplements include another compound to increase the absorbance. Of the various forms of zinc, the zinc glycinate and picolinate have the best absorption, so these are what I recommend. The typical dosage of zinc supplements is around 30 mg daily. A higher dosage can lead to low copper levels in your body so it's good to keep checking copper levels when taking zinc supplements. But overall zinc supplement is well tolerated and is important for reversing Hashimoto's disease.

Vitamin D: As mentioned, vitamin D is important for many different functions in our body, including the thyroid. Vitamin D helps with modulating our immune function and reducing inflammation, especially in Hashimoto's patients. Most people are low in vitamin D levels, so it is important to check your levels; the other challenge is knowing the optimal levels of vitamin D, as the range on blood work is very wide: 30 to 100 ng/ml. I feel the optimal levels of Vitamin D in people with Hashimoto's is anything more than 50ng/ml. For most people the ideal dosage is between 2,000 and 5,000 units daily, but I always recommend checking the levels before you start the supplement.

Magnesium: Magnesium is a mineral and is part of more than 300 enzymes in our body that help with various biochemical processes. Magnesium helps with the proper production of energy and is responsible for the production of DNA/RNA; it also helps with controlling the inflammation in the body.

In people with Hashimoto's, magnesium helps with iodine uptake in the thyroid gland and thyroid hormone production; it also reduces oxidative stress, especially in the thyroid gland. Low magnesium levels have been associated with immune dysfunction and also with high thyroid antibodies. Magnesium is involved in mitochondrial energy production and helps with the rejuvenation of mitochondria by controlling some of the repair mechanisms.

There are various supplement forms of magnesium, and the ideal form depends on other conditions the patient might have. For example, magnesium citrate helps if a patient has thyroid plus constipation issues. This form of magnesium keeps your bowels regular and also supports thyroid health. Another form of magnesium is magnesium glycinate, which is very relaxing. This can be taken in the evening and that helps with reducing stress, as well as supporting the thyroid. Generally, the dosage for both forms can be between 320 mg and 420 mg. The good news is that we don't see toxicity or other side effects from magnesium. Given this, I feel everyone with thyroid disorder should include a magnesium supplement on a daily basis.

Omega-3 fatty acids: The best way to fight the underlying inflammation that causes Hashimoto's is through the Omega 3 fatty acids EPA and DHA.

As we saw in the section on nutrition, Omega-3 fatty acids are very potent in reducing inflammation because they modulate the immune pathways. Omega-3 fatty acids have also shown particular benefits in improving brain function in thyroid conditions. It was seen in a research study on hypothyroid rats that when they were supplemented with Omega-3 fatty acids their brain functioning improved significantly. Also, Omega 3 are very good antioxidants and protect your mitochondria. They are also beneficial for chronic pain, fatigue, and improving cholesterol issues.

An important factor to consider is the source of your Omega-3 and also the dosage. The most common source of Omega-3 in supplementation is by taking fish oil capsules. There are few things we need to keep in mind when trying to take fish oil, such as where it was made. If not sourced properly it can be very high in mercury, and as we already know high levels of mercury can be detrimental to Hashimoto's patients. Another issue is that fish oil can get rancid very easily and is heat- sensitive, so most of the fish oil off the shelf is not providing any benefit. Even Amazon warehouses are not temperature controlled so you need to be careful where you buy it from.

The recommended dosage of Omega-3 is a minimum of between 2 and 3 grams daily. Now, this is where I have seen so many companies making fools of their consumers. The labels on fish oil supplements will claim there is more than 1000 mg of Omega's in one capsule. But when you read it carefully you will see that the actual Omega-3s, which are DHA and EPA, are far less than that. When you buy the Omega-3 supplement make sure you combine the amount of EPA and DHA and that it's more than 2 grams.

Vitamin B12

Supplementation of vitamin B12 is especially important in Hashimoto's patients because their bodies might not be able to absorb this vitamin through food. There are various forms of vitamin B12 which are available in supplement form, so it is very important to know which one is the best.

Most of the vitamin B12 supplements contain cyanocobalamin, but the better form is Methylcobalamin, as this is better absorbed and utilized by your body.

Vitamin B12 supplements are available as capsules, injections or sublingual pills. I feel sublingual and injectable forms are the best form of Vitamin B12 supplements because as mentioned some people with Hashimoto's might have problems absorbing vitamin B12 from their gut. In fact, a study showed equal efficacy of sublingual as compared to injectable vitamin B12. I generally recommend sublingual 1000mcg of vitamin B12 daily.

The injectable will have different dosages, generally around 1000 mcg once a week for the first month, then 1000mcg once a month.

CoQ10: This is one of the most important supplements needed for the mito-thyroid connection. CoQ10 is an important co-factor involved in mitochondrial functioning. It also acts as an antioxidant and helps protect the mitochondria from any kind of oxidative damage. There have been several studies which has shown improvement of mitochondrial function after taking this supplement. CoQ10 also has been associated with improving the vascularity of thyroid gland. Given all this, Co Q10 is very beneficial for Hashimoto's patients.

It also is very helping in treating fatigue and brain fog. Various forms of CoQ10 are available and they can have different absorption capacity. The dosage can vary greatly depending on the company but is generally between 30 and 90 mg per day.

Acetyl l Carnitine: Carnitine supplements became popular as they have shown to improve muscle strength and endurance significantly. In fact, several athletes and people in the fitness industry started taking this supplement and saw phenomenal results.

We have good research studies that show acetyl l carnitine supplement improves fatigue and brain fog, as well as muscle mass and performance. Acetyl l carnitine's role in our body is mainly the transportation of fatty acids into the mitochondria to help produce energy. It also acts as an antioxidant and helps to reduce the free radicals, thus protecting both our thyroid and mitochondria.

Acetyl carnitine can be helpful for both hyperthyroid and Hashimoto's patients, whose skeletal muscles tend to be low in carnitine. There was 2016 study in which patients with hypothyroidism were supplemented with carnitine and had significant improvement in their fatigue. I have seen significant improvement in Hashimoto's symptoms, especially brain fog, weakness and tiredness, after taking carnitine supplement. The typical dosage for Acetyl l carnitine is 1 to 2 grams daily.

CHAPTER 18

NANCY THE NAPPING
LADY RUNS A MARATHON

Recall Nancy, whose life was being ruined due to Hashimoto's-related fatigue. When Nancy came to see me she had lost all hope of getting better and she was even feeling that she was not a good mother to her children. Her quality of life was very poor and she was not able to do any of the things she loved, like running or hanging out with friends. The medicines were not working and she was struggling to get through each day.

After doing evaluations we figured that Nancy had several factors that were causing her to feel fatigued all the time, including MTHFR, adrenal dysfunction, and underlying inflammation. Out of all these things, the MTHFR was causing the biggest issue.

MTHFR is an enzyme that helps in the processing of folate (vitamin B9) in your body. The folate from the food needs to be converted to an active version (5-Methyltetrahydrofolate) so that your body can utilize it. In some people, there is a genetic mutation of the MTHFR gene that interferes with folate conversion. This has several downstream effects, one of which is that it interferes with the mito-thyroid connection. Mitochondrial health is compromised because of the MTHFR mutation and that leads to the development of symptoms like fatigue, brain fog, and mood changes.

Once we identified Nancy's problems we started her on the mito-thyroid diet, which provided her body with foods that were high in folate and B12, like green leafy vegetables. We also started her on a supplement regimen of methylated folate, methylated B12, and vitamin D, as well as CoQ10, carnitine, and alpha lipoic acid to provide mitochondrial support.

Within a few weeks of starting this regimen, Nancy saw a dramatic transformation. Her energy levels improved, the need to take naps disappeared, and she started participating in her kids' school activities again. This was huge for Nancy, and the first time she was able to attend her son's baseball game tears were rolling down her eyes. Nancy was able to get back to her exercising and now she is planning to run a marathon.

Nobody imagined that her fatigue could be related to a genetic disorder that is so common these days. But once the root cause was identified and she was able to address it, her life completely changed.

STEP 3 REMOVING
THE TOXICITIES

In the previous steps, we worked on regenerating your thyroid and rejuvenating your mitochondria using the Mito-Thyroid Diet and associated supplements. In this final step, we are going to work on ridding yourself of toxicities that are not allowing your mito-thyroid connection work properly.

We know that there are several toxins that hijack this mito-thyroid connection, including chemical substances, stress, and various infections you get exposed to in your lifetime. Each interferes with the proper functioning of your body, and together they create a huge burden on your immune function that ultimately leads to destruction of the mito-thyroid connection. Addressing these toxicities is key to reversing Hashimoto's, as they not only improve your current symptoms but safeguard your thyroid against future damage. In this step we optimize the various detox channels and build your immune system from ground up so these toxicities no longer affect your thyroid.

CHAPTER 19

REMOVING THE STRESS TOXICITY

We have already spoken about how stress can be detrimental to Hashimoto's patients. It destroys the mito-thyroid connection and leads to all the symptoms associated with it.

Initially, most of the patients I speak to about stress say they handle it easily. Still, I always insist on starting a de-stressing exercise, and invariably they later report it made a huge difference in their Hashimoto's symptoms.

Stress is not only the trigger of your Hashimoto's but is also responsible for the ongoing damage, so until we stop this damage to the mito-thyroid connection you are not going to feel better. Our society makes us feel that if we can't handle stress it's a sign of weakness, when in fact stress is a toxicity that our surrounding environment creates, often to the detriment of our mental and physical health. We will all get exposed to some kind of stress – in the workplace, in our relationships, with regard to our health, et cetera. The purpose of destressing exercises is to remove the negative health effects of stress on our bodies.

Here are a few tips and tricks that I have used in my practice to help with this problem. They are simple and can easily be incorporated into your daily routine.

1. **Deep Breathing:** Breathing exercises can be very helpful for relaxation and they work very quickly. When we are stressed out we tend to take shallow breaths, which actually causes us to get more anxious. Shallow breathing leads to increased blood pressure; it also reduces the amount of oxygen that gets delivered to your brain. Most of us don't even realize that we are taking shallow breaths unless we try to take a deep one.

   There are several benefits to deep breathing, but one of the most important ones is that it reduces the burden of stress on the body. Deep breathing activates our parasympathetic nervous system, which helps us to relax. It also it provides more oxygen to the brain so it helps with brain fog.

I use a simple deep breathing exercise, called the 4-7-8 method, that has helped several of my patients. First, you empty your lungs, then take in a slow, deep breath for four seconds. You hold this breath for 7 seconds, then very slowly exhale for the count of eight seconds. You can repeat this cycle three to four times and it will help you to relax and feel more centered. The good part about this method is that you can do it anywhere, and it takes just a few minutes. Start your day with some deep breathing exercises, then do a few more cycles at midday, and again before you go to bed.

2. Meditation: This practice has been around for millennia, but in recent years it has become especially popular because of its many health benefits, including stress reduction.

For Hashimoto's patients, meditation is helpful because it improves cortisol levels and sleep, decreases inflammation, and balances hormones. There are so many different kinds of meditation practices and all of them work, so long as you are persistent. I tell my patients is to simply follow the practice that resonates for them.

It's always good to start with a guided meditation, whether it is following a voice prompt or nature's sounds. It also never hurts to take some online courses or training, for meditation does have a learning curve.

I recommend that you start slow by meditating for a few minutes a day and then slowly increase over time.

Another tip I can offer you is don't overthink it. Just do your meditation without worrying whether you are doing it correctly or not. At first you will find yourself inundated with several thoughts – that's normal. And yes, it is uncomfortable to sit with your own thoughts silently for even a few minutes because we are so used to be overstimulated by noise and technology. The good news is you don't have to fight your thoughts, you just have to ignore them and focus on the voice/nature prompts. With practice, you will slowly but surely gain better control over your mind.

The last tip is to make sure you associate the meditation time with some other daily activity so that it becomes part of your life. For example, you might do it in the morning as soon as you wake up, before you even get out of your bed. I do a meditation practice every day called <u>Heartfulness</u> and I recommend that everyone try it as it is so easy to do. Other mobile apps that people have found useful are Insight Timer, Calm, and Headspace.

3. **Nature:** Being in nature has so many healing properties and health benefits. Research now shows that being outdoors increases your brain function, gives you more energy and reduces stress.

For Hashimoto's patients, being outdoors helps with reducing inflammation and cortisol levels. So get away from your computer or phone and get outside – whether it's just for a short walk during your break or spending the weekends hiking or picnicking with your family. You will soon find yourself feeling both revitalized and more relaxed.

If you have Hashimoto's disease, stress management is not a choice – it's a necessity. Each and every Hashimoto's patient I have seen has improved her symptoms by implementing these stress reduction techniques. Most people think that you need to spend hours and hours on these techniques when the truth is just a few minutes a day can change your life.

4. **Supplements**: There are also certain supplements that can be helpful in dealing with stress so it doesn't hurt our body. All too often people are prescribed Xanax and other anxiety meds, with are habit-forming, cause terrible side effects, and do nothing to prevent the

future attacks of stress – none of which is true of these supplements.

The main category of supplements that helps with stress management is called adaptogens. These adaptogenic herbs, which have been used for centuries in Ayurvedic and Chinese medicine, are very useful in reducing the effects of stress on the body, whether physical or emotional.

Research has time and again shown that these herbs help reduce inflammation, improve our immunity, and help reduce cortisol levels. And, I have seen, they are especially helpful for Hashimoto's patients and should be a part of their healing protocol.

- **Ashwagandha**: Ashwagandha has been used by Ayurvedic practitioners for more than 3,000 years. In fact, it is called the "Queen of Ayurveda" because of its numerous health benefits, including stress reduction. It also helps with depression and anxiety as well.

Ashwagandha also has been shown to reduce cortisol levels and improve energy levels, mitochondrial, brain function – all of which is especially important for Hashimoto's patients.

Research also shows that it reduces the inflammation markers in the body. So you see, this is truly a magical supplement that can be helpful for so many different things. It targets all the underlying root causes of Hashimoto's and is very well tolerated by most people, with no side effects.

Most of the time adding Ashwagandha at nighttime is beneficial, as it improves sleep and relieve any anxiety associated with it. The typical dosage you can start with is around 400 to 500 mg each evening.

- **Rhodiola Rosea:** This is another adaptogenic herb that has been used for centuries and has several health benefits. Rhodiola stimulates the nervous system and thus helps with mental clarity and reducing brain fog; it has also been shown to decrease depression, stress and anxiety. But the main reason Rhodiola is so popular is its ability to eliminate fatigue, which is a common, chronic problem for Hashimoto's patients.

I recommend taking Rhodiola in the morning so it can boost energy without interfering with your sleep. The dosage range is wide, but you can start with 400 to 500 mg a day.

Bacopa: Also known as Brahmi, this is another Ayurvedic medicine with several health benefits. Bacopa has been useful in improving brain function and attention span. As brain fog and ADHD symptoms are very common in Hashimoto's patients, this herb can be very useful.

There was also a research study done in hypothyroid rats where some were given bacopa along with thyroid medicine. That group had higher levels of thyroid hormones, and experienced an improvement in antioxidant levels in the thyroid. But the most exciting result for Hashimoto's patients is that bacopa protects the thyroid gland from further damage. The typical dosage is 400-500 mg/day.

There are several other adaptogenic herbs – tulsi, Siberian ginseng, reishi mushrooms, Schisandra, and maca, to name a few – each with its own benefits. It is not possible to review all the adaptogens in this book, but in terms of safety and their use in Hashimoto's patients, the above three are most beneficial.

As you see, there are various ways you can take care of stress and trauma, which is a key step in your Hashimoto's healing journey. Several of my clients have done other things to get their Hashimoto's under control, but often nobody has spoken to them about stress management. Again, pick a habit you enjoy and start very slowly, just a few minutes a day) and then scale it up. That, coupled with one of the adaptogenic herbs, will bring you amazing results.

CHAPTER 20

REMOVING
ENVIRONMENTAL TOXINS

We have previously spoken about various kinds of toxins like heavy metals and mold that cause destruction to the mito-thyroid connection. Now we need to work on removing these toxins from your system.

Our bodies have built-in detoxifying mechanisms, but due to the increasing number of toxins in our environment they can get overburdened and ultimately give up. For those with Hashimoto's, this is even more problematic because their detox channels are already not working perfectly and get overburdened more quickly than other people's. Because of this, we have to help them detox in a gentle, gradual way; going too fast is likely to cause an unpleasant reaction.

The first thing we need to do is to open up and optimize your existing detox channels.

Natural Ways to Detox

1. **Sweating.** Sweating has several health benefits, one of which is that it's a very potent way to rid yourself of

toxins such as Bisphenol A, Phthalates, Heavy metals, and mold toxins. This is why saunas have become very popular as a means of improving health. There are several kinds of saunas available, however, I feel infrared saunas offer more advantage than a regular sauna, as they use light to heat your body directly, instead of heating the air around you which in turn heats your body. This means with the infrared sauna you have deeper penetration and a better sweat.

Some tips about saunas:

I recommend that you shower immediately after being in the sauna, the reason being the toxins that are released through your skin will be washed off your body instead of being reabsorbed.

I also recommend starting off with a few minutes and slowly building up as tolerated, especially for people with Hashimoto's as some are unable to sweat and get super-heated in saunas.

2. **Through the GI tract:** Our gastrointestinal tract is an important channel of detoxification. Every bowel movement you have removes a certain amount of toxins from your body, so regular bowel movements are very important to our health. People who don't have regular bowel movements are more toxic because all those toxins that are supposed to be eliminated from the body through bowels get reabsorbed into the body. Some people take binder supplements, which bind toxins in the gastrointestinal tract and help eliminate them. However, what these people don't realize is that if you don't have regular bowel movements those binders will

not work. Several patients of mine had been told that not having daily bowel movements is normal for them, but I feel that at least one bowel movement a day is necessary for the body to rid itself of toxins.

Here are some tips on how to get regular bowel movements. Eating a fiber-rich diet that includes lots of vegetables is a must. Drink water on regular intervals throughout the day. If this doesn't work, add a fiber supplement like psyllium. Regular exercise also helps a lot of people to have regular bowel movements. One supplement that works in almost all of my patients is magnesium citrate, which promotes regularity and provides the daily magnesium requirement. If one pill doesn't work you can safely increase the dosage to get regular bowel movements.

3. **Kidneys:** Our kidneys filter our blood and get rid of various toxins that would otherwise accumulate in our system and ultimately cause several health issues. For our kidneys to work properly we need an adequate amount of water, but most of us don't drink enough during the day. Soft drinks, coffee or teas don't count! Another important thing to remember is that we have to spread out our water consumption throughout the day, not all in one go. On average, I feel everyone should drink at least eight to ten glasses of water daily but it can vary depending on then individual.

Tips about water intake: Most of my clients tell me that plain water doesn't taste good and that it is very boring. To make it more interesting you can add some lemon, cucumber, or a few drops of essential oil like sweet orange.

Another issue we face concerns the source of drinking water. I believe the best resource is filtered water. Water in plastic bottles may have been sitting on the shelf for several months and therefore contaminated with BPA or other toxins. But you also have to source the right filter, as the majority of the over the tap filters might not be good enough. Reverse osmosis filters are the best as they remove the majority of the toxins.

4. **Lymphatic System:** This is an under appreciated but essential channel of detoxification. The lymphatic system is part of our circulatory system and primarily transports lymph throughout our body. This lymph has various functions, the most important being modulating our immune function and helping to get rid of waste products and toxins from our body. One of the things that helps with lymph flow is muscle contractions, so many people will go for lymphatic massages. The other easy method for optimizing this detox channel is through something called dry brushing. Dry brushing is a method where you use a brush with stiff bristles and stroke your skin with it to help detox and open skin pores. The way to brush your skin is to move with the blood flow, starting at the periphery and moving towards the center. For example, start at your feet and then move upwards; do the same thing with your arms and move towards the center. It is simple and doesn't take too long (you can do before your shower), but is powerful for opening up your detox channels.

5. **Liver:** The liver plays a major role in several important bodily functions including digestion and storage; it is also our master detoxifier organ. The prevalence of liver

dysfunction, especially fatty liver, is very high in people with Hashimoto's. Most of the time the blood work will show the liver function to be normal, but there might still be dysfunction, as these tests don't tell us about all the liver's detox pathways. Luckily, there are several ways in which we can optimize liver function, for example with specific foods and supplements, so it can help your body to detox properly.

Food that support liver detox:

Cruciferous vegetables like broccoli, cauliflower, and Brussels sprouts support the liver, specifically due to compounds called sulforaphane. Artichokes protect the liver from damage and also support the production of bile, which again helps with detoxification. Adding green tea regularly to your diet also helps with detox, so I suggest at least 2 to 3 cups of organic green tea for my clients. These foods are already part of your Mito-thyroid Diet so you should be good, but for detox you can pay more attention to them.

Supplements to help detox

1. **N- acetyl cysteine (NAC).** NAC, which is a derivative of an amino acid in our body called cysteine, has various health benefits. In the conventional medical world, it is used to treat people with Tylenol (acetaminophen) toxicity, which it does by providing protection to the liver via the generation of glutathione and also by acting as an antioxidant. For our purposes here, however, it's important to know that NAC helps with detox. It has also been shown to be protective of mitochondria

and the thyroid and is therefore helpful for Hashimoto's patients. The general dosage of NAC is 500 mg twice daily.

2. **Milk Thistle:** Milk thistle is a very important detox supplement. It helps support the liver and has been used to treat liver diseases, especially fatty liver disease and cirrhosis. The active ingredient in milk thistle is called silymarin and it works to protect the liver by acting as an antioxidant, reducing inflammation, and supporting glutathione production. The general dosage of milk thistle is 140 mg, taken twice daily.

3. **Alpha lipoic acid (ALA):** ALA is another powerful antioxidant and detoxifier which can be helpful for Hashimoto's patients. It decreases inflammation in the body and is also helpful in detoxification of mycotoxins and heavy metals. Research has shown that ALA also reduces inflammatory markers in the liver and improves insulin resistance, which is a reason many people with Hashimoto's are not able to lose weight. One caution that I give my patients is to not take this supplement with thyroid medications, as it can interfere with their conversion. The general dosage of ALA is 500-600 mg daily.

4. **Curcumin:** Turmeric has been used as a spice and as a medicine for centuries now. In recent years we've come to know that the medicinal qualities are due to a compound called curcumin. Curcumin reduces inflammation, improves the oxidative capacity of the body, and helps support the detox system. Curcumin has been helpful in several autoimmune diseases, especially

rheumatoid arthritis. It is also very helpful in treating Hashimoto's disease because it positively influences our immune function and reduces the inflammatory markers like IL6 and TNF alpha, both of which have been associated with thyroid destruction. And, for females with thyroid nodules and thyroid cancer, it can be a life-savior.

Curcumin also has high antioxidant properties which protects both the thyroid and mitochondria. In mitochondria, curcumin not only reduces oxidative stress markers, but also helps with regeneration and regulates proper functioning. The antioxidant nature of curcumin protects the liver from any damage from various kinds of toxins. The most common dosage of curcumin is 1 to 2 grams daily.

CHAPTER 21

FREIDA'S JOURNEY FROM BRAIN FOG TO MENTAL CLARITY

Freida felt alone in this world when she was suffering from brain fog. None of the people around her even knew what brain fog was. She was also really worried that she would get dementia and end up in a nursing home. Initially, she thought her Hashimoto's might be causing it, but despite her hopes that the thyroid medicine would help, things continued to get worse.

After a thorough evaluation of Freida, I identified mold toxins in her body that were causing her brain fog symptoms. As we discussed before, mold toxins break the mito-thyroid connection, causing not only Hashimoto's but brain fog symptoms.

Frieda had moved into a new house four years ago, and a year later started having brain fog symptoms along with constant sinus drainage and allergies. She never suspected her house might be making her sick until she saw me and we put the two and two together. Suddenly it dawned on her that her basement did smell musty at times, but she never paid much attention to it. A simple urine test showed that she had high levels of mold toxins in her system.

We started her on a detox protocol by optimizing all the detox channels that we spoke about in the previous chapter. We also created a specific mold detox protocol that included a special diet and supplements. Initially, she didn't see much change (this is normal for patients with mold as it takes a while for the toxins to leave their body), but after a few months she got rid of the brain fog and felt her mental capacity improve drastically. Remember the notepad she had to carry to each business meeting? Well, she was now able to "forget" about it and focus on listening to her colleagues and clients.

Identifying the mold toxins and treating them brought a ray of light back in Freida's life. She went from worrying about dementia to having a memory just as sharp as a much younger person.

CHAPTER 22

REMOVING INFECTIONS TO STRENGTHEN IMMUNITY

We now turn to how we can rid of the viruses, parasites, and other pathogens that may have caused your Hashimoto's disease and are exacerbating your symptoms. Remember, most of these infections have passed the acute phase to become chronic.

The most important thing you can do to help your body deal with these pathogens is to keep your immune system healthy. Here are some things you can start incorporating into your life right away.

Lifestyle Changes to improve immunity

1. Food: A clean diet is the foundation of a good and healthy immune system. The Mito-Thyroid diet I recommend in this book includes all the foods that help to rebuild your immunity, such as clean protein, good fats, and rainbow vegetables. It also eliminates foods that suppress your immune system like sugar, gluten, dairy, soy, and corn. As mentioned, if you follow this diet you

will reap many benefits for your thyroid, one of them being keeping your immunity in good shape.

2. Sleep: Getting enough good quality sleep is also key to a healthy immune system. Most people think sleep is only good to repair your body and to give it a break. While this is true, the research shows that sleep also helps to rebuild your immunity. During sleep, we produce chemicals called cytokines, which help our immune system fight infections and stay healthy. When our sleep is poor, our body doesn't produce these cytokines, which leads to weak immunity. Sleep also helps other immune cells in our body called T cells. In sleep-deprived individuals the T cells do not function as effectively, which also affects their ability to fight infections. Unfortunately, the majority of people (70% in the U.S.) don't get enough sleep and therefore have compromised immune systems. I recommend that everyone get at least eight hours of sleep every night. Remember, though, quality is as important as quantity. Some tips that can help you to get good quality sleep are:

- Create a sleep routine: you go to sleep at the same time and in the same place.

- No screen activity for at least 1 hour before bedtime.

- No caffeinated beverages in the evening.

- Use blue light-blocking glasses as soon as the sun goes down so that your melatonin (the sleep hormone) secretion doesn't get affected and you can get good sleep.

3. Stress: We have discussed how stress management is so important for your thyroid. Here I want to show the importance of stress management to rejuvenate your immunity. Stress is a killer of our immune system. Chronic stress leads to HPA axis (hypothalamic–pituitary–adrenal) dysfunction and leads to excessive production of cortisol, which suppresses our natural defenses. Chronic stress also affects your sympathetic nervous system by taking control of the lymphoid system, which also decreases immunity. It is during stressful times that our immune system gets weak and underlying infections get reactivated, which can lead to Hashimoto's. We have already spoken about simple things you can do like deep breathing and meditation to manage stress. Supplements like ashwagandha can also be very helpful and actually have been shown to improve immunity.

4. Gut health: Who would have thought one hundred years ago that the gut is the most important immune system regulator in our body? Back then, we only associated the gut with the digestion of food and absorbing nutrients. However, in recent years we have realized that it plays a critical role in our overall heath and ability to fight off threats.

   The majority (70-80%) of the immune cells in our body are located in the gut. We have an estimated 100 trillion bacteria living there as well. (We actually have ten times more bacterial cells in our body than we have our own cells.) For millions of years now we have been developing a symbiotic relationship with this bacteria and our body's immune system has evolved along it.

A healthy microbiome supports our immune system by supporting the development of immune cells and also controls the functioning of these immune cells; therefore, taking care of this microbiome is of the utmost importance. Research has shown that people with a poor microbiome in their gut also have poor immune systems.

There are several ways to keep your microbiome in good health, but the two most important ones are prebiotics and probiotics. Now, most of you might have heard about probiotics but not so much about prebiotics. Prebiotics are basically food for your good bacteria and promotes its growth.

Prebiotics are typically different kinds of fiber derivatives that are resistant to enzymatic and chemical digestion in our gut until they reach the large intestine. Once there, the fermentation of these prebiotic fibers happens by good bacteria which leads to the production of fatty acids (SCFA) like acetate, butyrate, and propionate. These SCFA play an important role in modulating our gut's immunity and helps in reducing inflammation too. Prebiotic- rich foods include onions, artichokes, chicory root, garlic, apple, asparagus, and dandelion, so make an effort to include these foods regularly in your diet.

Another way to keep your gut microbiome in good shape is through probiotics. Probiotics are basically a collection of good bacteria which keep our immune system healthy. Some of the probiotic foods that are healthy for Hashimoto's patients are sauerkraut, kimchi, dairy-free yogurt, and kombucha.

Supplements to improve immunity and fight infections

Along with lifestyle changes, there are several supplements that can help your immune system become healthy. It is important to know that the supplements we are talking about here are *not* for the acute treatment of infections. These are more so to keep your immune system healthy so your body is able to fight chronic infections more effectively. That said, there are several chronic infections like certain parasites, Lyme, et cetera that will need more elaborate protocols to treat them completely. For that you need to see a trained Functional Medicine physician.

Now let's talk about immune-boosting supplements that most people with Hashimoto's will need to keep their immune system healthy and thus safeguard their thyroid from further autoimmune damage.

1. **Vitamin C:** Vitamin C is a potent antioxidant and has multiple health benefits attached to it — including the improvement of our immunity. Vitamin C modulates cellular defense and viral-induced processes in our body, which helps us fight chronic viral infections. A Cochrane Review was done to evaluate whether vitamin C is useful in treating the common cold and concluded that it indeed decreases the symptoms. Along with helping your body to fight against viral infections, vitamin C also helps with reducing inflammation in the thyroid gland.

   I generally recommend using buffered vitamin C as that decreases the GI discomfort which a high dose can cause. Otherwise, there are no apparent side effects of vitamin C and it is water soluble so there is no concern of toxicity. The recommended dose is 2 to 3 grams daily, taken at different times.

2. **Probiotics:** We have discussed how probiotics keep our gut health – and thus our immunity – in good shape. It has shown that probiotic supplements interact with existing bacteria in our gut and helps secretions of chemokines and cytokines and regulate the function of T cells, B cells, dendritic cells, and macrophages, which improves our immunity. There are different kinds of probiotics available, but the most beneficial are the ones which have lactobacillus and Bifidobacterium species. The probiotic supplement should have at least 10 trillion bacterial strains in them.

3. **Vitamin D:** We have already discussed the importance for vitamin D, but I wanted to bring it up again to emphasize the importance of this vitamin for the thyroid. In addition to its many other health benefits, vitamin D helps our immune system by activating macrophages, stimulating antimicrobial peptides, and modulating TH17 cells and TGF beta. Most people think they are getting enough vitamin D from milk or sunlight, but in reality, all of us are deficient in Vitamin D until we take supplements. The recommended dosage is 5,000 units daily.

4. **Zinc:** As discussed previously, this is an important supplement for people with Hashimoto's as it helps with thyroid hormone production. But Zinc is also important

for keeping the immune system in good shape as it regulates the T-cell immune function; in fact, even a mild zinc deficiency can cause impairment of the immune system. A randomized, prospective study of over 1,600 infants under age two who received zinc supplementation showed decreased rates of pneumonia. A Cochrane database review and a trial in the Annals of Internal Medicine showed that zinc supplementation reduced the duration of the common cold. Different forms of zinc supplements are available, but the best form is zinc picolinate or zinc glycinate. The dosage is 30 to 60 mg daily.

5. **Omega 3 Supplements.** The two Omega-3 fatty acids that are essential for our body are EPA and DHA. These are important for the proper functioning of our immune system too. Omega-3 fatty acids are components of our cell membranes and regulate several properties of these membranes. They also act as signaling molecules and are involved in the activation of the immune system. Omega-3 fatty acids reduce the inflammation in our body and also boost immune cells and thus maintain a healthy balance of the immune system. Studies have shown that Omega-3 fatty acids can activate B cells and T cells and can also support other immune cells like macrophages to help supports the body's immunity. A word of caution here: be careful about which Omega-3 supplement you take as some are high in mercury. The dosage is generally between 2 to 3 grams daily of combined EPA and DHA.

The above lifestyle factors and supplements can help you to lay the foundation of a healthy immune system that can fight off the chronic infections your body has been dealing with. I know this to be true, as they have helped several of my patients in this situation. These infections were not letting their Hashimoto's heal, but once they did this protocol they saw phenomenal results.

As mentioned previously, sometimes you will need more advanced treatment for chronic infections like EBV, parasites, candida and Lyme disease. The advanced protocols must be carefully monitored by a trained Functional Medicine provider, for if not used properly they can cause significant reactions.

CHAPTER 23

WRAPPING IT UP

My primary purpose in writing this book was to let you know that you don't have to suffer because of Hashimoto's. There is hope for you to get better and improve your life.

As we have seen, Hashimoto's is a disease that affects every aspect of your life and it is not easy to live with it. We have also seen that, for many people, conventional medicine doesn't offer a solution. They are just given a pill and told there is nothing else to be done. Sometimes they are even blamed for their situation. As I have shown you, that is not the case; there is so much research out there about other things you can do to get better, and more studies are being done all the time.

Remember, the cause of your Hashimoto's symptoms – including weight gain, fatigue, brain fog, hair issues, and gut problems – is the broken connection between the thyroid gland and the mitochondria in your cells.

As mentioned in the first section, there are many triggers responsible for breaking this connection, such as food sensitivity, nutritional deficiency, toxins, and infections.

Once you've uncovered your triggers, the next section is to work on fixing this mito-thyroid connection. As discussed, proper nutrition is a powerful means of doing so, such as the Mito-thyroid diet I developed specially with Hashimoto's patients in mind. This diet not only helps in regenerating your thyroid but also rejuvenates your mitochondria, aids in detoxification, and builds your immunity. This diet alone has helped several of my clients get rid of their Hashimoto's symptoms. We also add supplements that support the healing process.

Once your mito-thyroid connection is healing we need to make sure that we get rid of toxicities that got you into this position in the first place. Each must be dealt with separately so your thyroid heals completely and that in the future your body is better prepared to protect it.

By following this three-step plan, you can regain your lost energy and focus, and you will feel lighter, happier and healthier than you have in a long time.

Future Steps: What happens if you are still not better?

This book covers the majority of the things that can help your Hashimoto's, but there are some people who need advanced intervention, such as:

1. LDN (Low-Dose Naltrexone). Naltrexone in high doses is typically used to treat people with opioid addiction. But researchers have noticed that a very low dose of this medicine is beneficial for autoimmune conditions, especially Hashimoto's. This new modality of treatment is promising and can be considered if patients are not getting better.

2. Peptides: These are specific sequences of amino acids that are naturally produced in the body. These peptides have far-reaching health effects as they bind to specific receptors in our cells and help the body to make positive health changes. Peptides are showing promising results in various health conditions, especially autoimmune diseases. I have helped several of my Hashimoto's patients using peptides, especially thymosin alpha 1; thymosin beta 4; and BPC 157, with phenomenal results. But it is important to work with a health professional with the right knowledge of these peptides so you don't do more harm than good.

3. Genetics: Thanks to technology, we have been able to map our entire genome; we can also use this genetic information to optimize health. Patients with Hashimoto's clients have several genetic problems that need to be evaluated, including MTHFR (which is a genetic mutation), a weakened detoxification system, gluten sensitivity, et cetera. By identifying these issues we can make a more specific plan that is required by your body to get better.

4. Mold and heavy metal detox: We have discussed previously how mold and heavy metals like mercury and lead can cause Hashimoto's. Some people's detox systems are not functioning appropriately and they need a more specific and vigorous protocol to get rid of these toxins. For that, you will have to work with a qualified professional who has training and experience in this area.

5. Treat Underlying Infections. Sometimes getting rid of chronic infections like candida, EBV and Lyme disease

requires advanced protocols. These protocols are complicated and most physicians, even those who practice Functional Medicine, may not know the best way to treat them. If you are not getting better, don't give up until you find the right practitioner.

I have helped several Hashimoto's clients to get better by using these advanced protocols. If you need my help to get your Hashimoto's under control, you can get in touch with me at www.anshulguptamd.com

Here's What You Need to Do Next

This book has introduced you to the roadmap of recovery from Hashimoto's.

The next step in your healing journey is my 6-week Thyroid Reset Course. In this course I give you a complete game plan which tells you exactly what to do each week to improve your thyroid function.

You are provided with weekly checklists, handouts, recipes and self-assessment tools to keep you accountable and to succeed in reaching your health goals.

With this course you also get an option to work with me 1:1 to guide you during the implementation process.

To get more information about the course visit anshulguptamd.com/thyroidcourse

ABOUT THE AUTHOR

D r. Anshul Gupta is a speaker, author, researcher and a world expert in Hashimoto's disease. He educates people worldwide on reversing their Hashimoto's condition.

He is a Board-Certified Family Medicine Physician, with advanced certification in Functional Medicine, Peptide Therapy, and also Fellowship trained in Integrative Medicine.

He has worked at the prestigious Cleveland Clinic Department of Functional Medicine alongside Dr. Mark Hyman. He has helped thousands of patients to reverse their health issues by using the concepts of functional medicine.

His dedication towards his patients was recognized when he was awarded Readers' Choice, Best Doctor in Northern Neck Area.

He is now on a mission to help one million people reverse their health conditions. To achieve this mission, he has started a virtual functional medicine practice, a blog, and video series so he can reach people from all over the world.

Through his innovative approach towards Hashimoto's disease, he has helped several patients to reverse their unresolved symptoms and live their life to the fullest.

He loves to spend time with his wife and two kids. In his free time, he enjoys traveling, hiking in the woods, or meditating in a quiet spot.

You can know more about him at AnshulguptaMD.com

Social Media:

Instagram: https://www.instagram.com/anshulguptamd/

Youtube: https://www.youtube.com/c/AnshulGuptaMD

Linkedin: https://www.linkedin.com/in/anshulguptamd/

ACKNOWLEDGMENT

The journey of writing this book has been a long one; it began the day I started having my own health issues. This book is the culmination of efforts from all these years, and several people who have helped me during this journey.

First of all, my wife Kanwal has played a pivotal role in supporting me during my tough times. She encouraged me to write this book and was there whenever I needed her.

My thanks also goes to my parents and my two children who continue to inspire me to be better.

I learned a lot of about Functional Medicine through my mentors at Cleveland Clinic, especially Dr. Mark Hyman, Dr. Elizabeth Bradley and Dr. Alice Sullivan. They have all helped me to deepen my understanding of chronic diseases, which helped me to write this book.

I wanted to specially thank JJ. Virgin for helping me brainstorm the basic concept of this book. To Dana Micheli for her intensive editing work on this book. And to Shanda Trofe who helped me with all the publishing needs.

And thank you to all my patients, who have helped me to grow as a person and as a physician. You keep me motivated every day to keep going and keep getting better.

REFERENCES

1. Lahera V, de Las Heras N, López-Farré A, Manucha W, Ferder L. Role of Mitochondrial Dysfunction in Hypertension and Obesity. Curr Hypertens Rep. 2017;19(2):11. doi:10.1007/s11906-017-0710-9

2. Mercer JR, Yu E, Figg N, et al. The mitochondria-targeted antioxidant MitoQ decreases features of the metabolic syndrome in ATM+/-/ApoE-/- mice. Free Radic Biol Med. 2012;52(5):841-849. doi:10.1016/j.freeradbiomed.2011.11.026

3. Bournat JC, Brown CW. Mitochondrial dysfunction in obesity. Curr Opin Endocrinol Diabetes Obes. 2010;17(5):446-452. doi:10.1097/MED.0b013e32833c3026

4. Woo CY, Jang JE, Lee SE, Koh EH, Lee KU. Mitochondrial Dysfunction in Adipocytes as a Primary Cause of Adipose Tissue Inflammation. Diabetes Metab J. 2019;43(3):247-256. doi:10.4093/dmj.2018.0221

5. Schroeder Amy, Privalsky Martin. Thyroid Hormones, T3 and T4, in the Brain. Frontiers in Endocrinology . 2014; Vol 4.

6. Jeremy W.SmithA.TudorEvans et al. Thyroid hormones, brain function and cognition: a brief review. Neuroscience & Biobehavioral Reviews. Volume 26, Issue 1, January 2002, Pages 45-60

7. Belenguer P, Duarte JMN, Schuck PF, Ferreira GC. Mitochondria and the Brain: Bioenergetics and Beyond. Neurotox Res. 2019;36(2):219-238. doi:10.1007/s12640-019-00061-7

8. Grimm A, Eckert A. Brain aging and neurodegeneration: from a mitochondrial point of view. *J Neurochem.* 2017;143(4):418-431. doi:10.1111/jnc.14037

9. Modi HR, Katyare SS. Cadmium exposure-induced alterations in the lipid/phospholipids composition of rat brain microsomes and mitochondria. *Neurosci Lett.* 2009;464(2):108-112. doi:10.1016/j.neulet.2009.08.003

10. Beghoul A, Kebieche M, Gasmi S, et al. Impairment of mitochondrial integrity and redox status in brain regions during a low-dose long-term exposition of rats to pyrethrinoïds: the preventive effect of quercetin. *Environ Sci Pollut Res Int.* 2017;24(24):19714-19722. doi:10.1007/s11356-017-9675-0

11. Myhill S, Booth NE, McLaren-Howard J. Chronic fatigue syndrome and mitochondrial dysfunction. *Int J Clin Exp Med.* 2009;2(1):1-16.

12. Behan WMH, More IAR, Behan PO. Mitochondrial abnormalities in the postviral fatigue syndrome. *Acta Neuropathol (Berl)* 1991;83:61–65

13. Fulle S, Mecocci P, Fano G, Vecchiet I, Vecchini A, Racciotti D, Cherubini A, Pizzigallo E, Vecchiet L, Senin U, Beal MF. Specific oxidative alterations in vastus lateralis muscle of patients with the diagnosis of chronic fatigue syndrome. *Free Radic Biol Med.* 2000;29:1252-1259.

14. Plioplys AV, Plioplys S. Serum levels of carnitine in chronic fatigue syndrome: clinical correlates. *Neuropsychobiology.* 1995;32:132–138.

15. Carroccio A, et al. (2015). High proportions of people with non-celiac wheat sensitivity have autoimmune disease or antinuclear antibodies. DOI:10.1053/j.gastro.2015.05.040

16. Matana A, Torlak V etal. Dietary Factors Associated with Plasma Thyroid Peroxidase and Thyroglobulin Antibodies.Nutrients. 2017 Oct 28;9(11). pii: E1186. doi: 10.3390/nu9111186.

17. Sachmechi I, Khalid A etal. Autoimmune Thyroiditis with Hypothyroidism Induced by Sugar Substitutes.. Cureus. 2018 Sep 7;10(9):e3268. doi: 10.7759/cureus.3268

18. Picca A, Riezzo G, Lezza AMS, et al. Mitochondria and redox balance in coeliac disease: A case-control study. Eur J Clin Invest. 2018;48(2):10.1111/eci.12877. doi:10.1111/eci.12877

19. Arikawa AY, Jakits HE, Flood A, et al. Consumption of a high glycemic load but not a high glycemic index diet is marginally associated with oxidative stress in young women. Nutr Res. 2015;35(1):7-13. doi:10.1016/j.nutres.2014.10.005

20. Rizwan H, Pal S, Sabnam S, Pal A. High glucose augments ROS generation regulates mitochondrial dysfunction and apoptosis via stress signalling cascades in keratinocytes. Life Sci. 2020;241:117148. doi:10.1016/j.lfs.2019.117148

21. Kahrizi F, Salimi A, Noorbakhsh F, et al. Repeated Administration of Mercury Intensifies Brain Damage in Multiple Sclerosis through Mitochondrial Dysfunction. Iran J Pharm Res. 2016;15(4):834-841.

22. Carocci A, Rovito N, Sinicropi MS, Genchi G. Mercury toxicity and neurodegenerative effects. Rev Environ Contam Toxicol. 2014;229:1-18. doi:10.1007/978-3-319-03777-6_1

23. Joel N. Meyer, Maxwell C. K. Leung, John P. Rooney, Ataman Sendoel, Michael O. Hengartner, Glen E. Kisby, Amanda S. Bess, Mitochondria as a Target of Environmental Toxicants, Toxicological Sciences, Volume 134, Issue 1, July 2013, Pages 1–17

24. Sousa CA, Soares EV. Mitochondria are the main source and one of the targets of Pb (lead)-induced oxidative stress in the yeast Saccharomyces cerevisiae. Appl Microbiol Biotechnol. 2014;98(11):5153-5160. doi:10.1007/s00253-014-5631-9

25. Winzelberg GG, Gore J, Yu D, Vagenakis AG, Braverman LE. Aspergillus flavus as a cause of thyroiditis in an immunosuppressed host. Johns Hopkins Med J. 1979 Mar;144(3):90-3.

26. Allan Lieberman, Luke Curtis. Mold Exposure and Mitochondrial Antibodies. Altern Ther Health Med.2020 Feb 21;AT5799.

27. Taija Liisa Somppi. Non-Thyroidal Illness Syndrome in Patients Exposed to Indoor Air Dampness Microbiota Treated Successfully with Triiodothyronine. Front Immunol. 2017; 8: 919.

28. Leemans M, Couderq S, Demeneix B, Fini JB. Pesticides With Potential Thyroid Hormone-Disrupting Effects: A Review of Recent Data. Front Endocrinol (Lausanne). 2019;10:743. Published 2019 Dec 9. doi:10.3389/fendo.2019.00743

29. Goldner WS, Sandler DP, Yu F, Hoppin JA, Kamel F, Levan TD. Pesticide use and thyroid disease among women in the Agricultural Health Study. Am J Epidemiol. 2010;171(4):455-464. doi:10.1093/aje/kwp404

30. Bailey DC, Todt CE, Burchfield SL, et al. Chronic exposure to a glyphosate-containing pesticide leads to mitochondrial dysfunction and increased reactive oxygen species production in Caenorhabditis elegans. Environ Toxicol Pharmacol. 2018;57:46-52. doi:10.1016/j.etap.2017.11.005

31. Peixoto F. Comparative effects of the Roundup and glyphosate on mitochondrial oxidative phosphorylation. Chemosphere. 2005 Dec;61(8):1115-1122. DOI: 10.1016/j. chemosphere.2005.03.044.

32. Costa LG, de Laat R, Tagliaferri S, Pellacani C. A mechanistic view of polybrominated diphenyl ether (PBDE) developmental neurotoxicity. Toxicol Lett. 2014;230(2):282-294. doi:10.1016/j.toxlet.2013.11.011

33. Turyk ME, Persky VW, Imm P, Knobeloch L, Chatterton R, Anderson HA. Hormone disruption by PBDEs in adult male sport fish consumers. Environ Health Perspect. 2008 Dec;116(12):1635-41. doi: 10.1289/ehp.11707. Epub 2008 Jul 24. PMID: 19079713; PMCID: PMC2599756.

34. Moon MK, Kim MJ, Jung IK, et al. Bisphenol A impairs mitochondrial function in the liver at doses below the no observed adverse effect level. J Korean Med Sci. 2012;27(6):644-652. doi:10.3346/jkms.2012.27.6.644

35. Khan S, Beigh S, Chaudhari BP, et al. Mitochondrial dysfunction induced by Bisphenol A is a factor of its hepatotoxicity in rats. Environ Toxicol. 2016;31(12):1922-1934. doi:10.1002/tox.22193

36. Choi EM, Suh KS, Rhee SY, et al. Perfluorooctanoic acid induces mitochondrial dysfunction in MC3T3-E1 osteoblast cells. J Environ Sci Health A Tox Hazard Subst Environ Eng. 2017;52(3):281-289. doi:10.1080/10934529.2016.1253402

37. Chaudhuri A, Koner S. A study of correlation of perceived stress and thyroid function among females in a rural population of reproductive age group. Med J DY Patil Vidyapeeth 2020;13:30-6.

38. Mizokami T, Wu Li A, El-Kaissi S, Wall JR. Stress and thyroid autoimmunity. Thyroid. 2004 Dec;14(12):1047-55. doi: 10.1089/thy.2004.14.1047. PMID: 15650357.

39. Fischer S, Strahler J, Markert C, Skoluda N, Doerr JM, Kappert M, Nater UM. Effects of acute psychosocial stress on the hypothalamic-pituitary-thyroid (HPT) axis in healthy women. Psychoneuroendocrinology. 2019 Dec;110:104438. doi: 10.1016/j.psyneuen.2019.104438. Epub 2019 Sep 6. PMID: 31563038.

40. Bagnasco M, Bossert I, Pesce G. Stress and autoimmune thyroid diseases. Neuroimmunomodulation. 2006;13(5-6):309-17. doi: 10.1159/000104859. Epub 2007 Aug 6. PMID: 17709953.

41. Picard M, McEwen BS. Psychological Stress and Mitochondria: A Systematic Review. *Psychosom Med*. 2018;80(2):141-153. doi:10.1097/PSY.0000000000000545

42. Xu B, Lang LM, Li SZ, Guo JR, Wang JF, Wang D, Zhang LP, Yang HM, Lian S. Cortisol Excess-Mediated Mitochondrial Damage Induced Hippocampal Neuronal Apoptosis in Mice Following Cold Exposure. Cells. 2019 Jun 18;8(6):612. doi: 10.3390/cells8060612. PMID: 31216749; PMCID: PMC6627841.

43. Picard, Martin PhD; McEwen, Bruce S. PhD Psychological Stress and Mitochondria: A Conceptual Framework, Psychosomatic Medicine: 2/3 2018 - Volume 80 - Issue 2 - p 126-140 doi: 10.1097/PSY.0000000000000544

44. Davies TF. Infection and autoimmune thyroid disease. J Clin Endocrinol Metab 2008; 93: 674–676.

45. Tomer Y, Davies TF. Infection, thyroid disease, and autoimmunity. Endocr Rev. 1993;14(1):107-120. doi:10.1210/edrv-14-1-107

46. Cusick MF, Libbey JE, Fujinami RS. Molecular mimicry as a mechanism of autoimmune disease. Clin Rev Allergy Immunol. 2012;42(1):102-111. doi:10.1007/s12016-011-8294-7

47. Janegova A, Janega P, Rychly B, Kuracinova K, Babal P. The role of Epstein-Barr virus infection in the development of autoimmune thyroid diseases. Endokrynol Pol. 2015;66(2):132-136. doi:10.5603/EP.2015.0020

48. Vernon SD, Whistler T, Cameron B, Hickie IB, Reeves WC, Lloyd A. Preliminary evidence of mitochondrial dysfunction associated with post-infective fatigue after acute infection with Epstein Barr virus. BMC Infect Dis. 2006;6:15. Published 2006 Jan 31. doi:10.1186/1471-2334-6-15

49. Khan M, Syed GH, Kim SJ, Siddiqui A. Mitochondrial dynamics and viral infections: A close nexus. Biochim Biophys Acta. 2015;1853(10 Pt B):2822-2833. doi:10.1016/j.bbamcr.2014.12.040

50. Rajič B1, Arapović J. Eradication of Blastocystis hominis prevents the development of symptomatic Hashimoto's thyroiditis: a case report.J Infect Dev Ctries. 2015 Jul 30;9(7):788-91. doi: 10.3855/jidc.4851.

51. El-Zawawy HT1, Farag HF. Improving Hashimoto's thyroiditis by eradicating Blastocystis hominis: Relation to IL-17.Ther Adv Endocrinol Metab. 2020 Feb 21;11:2042018820907013. doi: 10.1177/2042018820907013. eCollection 2020.

52. Benvenga, S., Guarneri, F. Molecular mimicry and autoimmune thyroid disease. Rev Endocr Metab Disord 17, 485–498 (2016). https://doi.org/10.1007/s11154-016-9363-2

53. COLEMAN, R. and HAY, R. (1997), Chronic mucocutaneous candidosis associated with hypothyroidism: a distinct syndrome?. British Journal of Dermatology, 136: 24-29. https://doi.org/10.1046/j.1365-2133.1997.d01-1137.x

54. Myhre, A.G., Stray-Pedersen, A., Spangen, S. et al. Chronic mucocutaneous candidiasis and primary hypothyroidism in two families. Eur J Pediatr 163, 604–611 (2004). https://doi.org/10.1007/s00431-004-1516-8

55. Vojdani A, Rahimian P, Kalhor H, Mordechai E. Immunological cross reactivity between Candida albicans and human tissue. Journal of Clinical & Laboratory Immunology. 1996 ;48(1):1-15.

56. Gürsoy S, Koçkar T, Atik SU, Önal Z, Önal H, Adal E. Autoimmunity and intestinal colonization by Candida albicans in patients with type 1 diabetes at the time of the diagnosis. Korean J Pediatr. 2018;61(7):217-220. doi:10.3345/kjp.2018.61.7.217

57. Singh SK, Girschick HJ. Lyme borreliosis: from infection to autoimmunity. Clin Microbiol Infect. 2004;10(7):598-614. doi :10.1111/j.1469-0691.2004.00895.

58. Davis DR, Epp MD, Riordan HD. Changes in USDA food composition data for 43 garden crops, 1950 to 1999. J Am Coll Nutr. 2004;23(6):669-682. doi:10.1080/07315724.2004.10719409

59. Schomburg L. Selenium, selenoproteins and the thyroid gland: interactions in health and disease. Nature Reviews Endocrinology. 2012;8(3):160–171. doi: 10.1038/nrendo.2011.174.

60. Saranac L., Zivanovic S., Bjelakovic B., Stamenkovic H., Novak M., Kamenov B. Why is the thyroid so prone to autoimmune disease? Hormone Research in Pædiatrics. 2011;75(3):157–165. doi: 10.1159/000324442.

61. Selenium and the thyroid gland: more good news for clinicians. Drutel A, Archambeaud F, Caron P. Clin Endocrinol (Oxf). 2013 Feb; 78(2):155-64.

62. Selenium and human health.Rayman MP. Lancet. 2012 Mar 31; 379(9822):1256-68.

63. Selenium: an element for life.Duntas LH, Benvenga S. Endocrine. 2015 Apr; 48(3):756-75.

64. Derumeaux H, Valeix P, Castetbon K, Bensimon M, Boutron-Ruault MC, Arnaud J, Hercberg S. Association of selenium with thyroid volume and echostructure in 35- to 60-year-old French adults. Eur J Endocrinol 2003;148(3):309-15.

65. Rasmussen LB, Schomburg L, Kohrle J, Pedersen IB, Hollenbach B, Hog A, et al. Selenium status, thyroid volume, and multiple nodule formation in an area with mild iodine deficiency. Eur J Endocrinol 2011;164:585-90.

66. Selenium supplementation in patients with autoimmune thyroiditis decreases thyroid peroxidase antibodies concentrations. Gärtner R, Gasnier BC, Dietrich JW, Krebs B, Angstwurm MWJ Clin Endocrinol Metab. 2002 Apr; 87(4):1687-91.

67. Effects of a six-month treatment with selenomethionine in patients with autoimmune thyroiditis.Duntas LH, Mantzou E, Koutras DA. Eur J Endocrinol. 2003 Apr; 148(4):389-93.

68. Selenium in the treatment of autoimmune thyroiditis. Gärtner R, Gasnier BC. Biofactors. 2003; 19(3-4):165-70.

69. Predicted dietary intake of selenium by the general adult population in Belgium.Waegeneers N, Thiry C, De Temmerman L, Ruttens A. Food Addit Contam Part A Chem Anal Control Expo Risk Assess. 2013; 30(2):278-85.

70. Selenium treatment in autoimmune thyroiditis: 9-month followup with variable doses..Turker O, Kumanlioglu K, Karapolat I, Dogan I. J Endocrinol. 2006 Jul; 190(1):151-6.

71. Institute of Medicine, Food and Nutrition Board. Dietary Reference Intakes: Vitamin C, Vitamin E, Selenium, and Carotenoids. National Academy Press, Washington, DC, 2000.

72. Burk RF, Norsworthy BK, Hill KE, Motley AK, Byrne DW. Effects of chemical form of selenium on plasma biomarkers in a high-dose human supplementation trial. Cancer Epidemiol Biomarkers Prev 2006;15:804-10

73. Perkins, Anthony & Fisher, Joshua & Vanderlelie, Jessica. (2016). Role of Selenium and Selenoproteins in mitochondrial function and disease. 10.18143/JISANH_v3i5_2059.

74. Mehta, S.L., Kumari, S., Mendelev, N. et al. Selenium preserves mitochondrial function, stimulates mitochondrial biogenesis, and reduces infarct volume after focal cerebral ischemia. BMC Neurosci 13, 79 (2012).

75. Severo JS1, Morais JBS The Role of Zinc in Thyroid Hormones Metabolism.Int J Vitam Nutr Res. 2019 Jul;89(1-2):80-88. doi: 10.1024/0300-9831/a000262. Epub 2019 Apr 15.

76. Mahmoodianfard S1, Vafa M2 Effects of Zinc and Selenium Supplementation on Thyroid Function in Overweight and Obese Hypothyroid Female Patients: A Randomized Double-Blind Controlled Trial.J Am Coll Nutr. 2015;34(5):391-9. doi: 10.1080/07315724.2014.926161. Epub 2015 Mar 11.

77. Costello LC, Franklin RB, Feng P. Mitochondrial function, zinc, and intermediary metabolism relationships in normal

prostate and prostate cancer. Mitochondrion. 2005;5(3):143-153. doi:10.1016/j.mito.2005.02.001

78. Yang, X., Wang, H., Huang, C. et al. Zinc enhances the cellular energy supply to improve cell motility and restore impaired energetic metabolism in a toxic environment induced by OTA. Sci Rep 7, 14669 (2017).

79. Chung HR. Iodine and thyroid function. Ann Pediatr Endocrinol Metab. 2014;19(1):8-12. doi:10.6065/apem.2014.19.1.8

80. Markou K, Georgopoulos N, Kyriazopoulou V, Vagenakis AG. Iodine-Induced hypothyroidism. Thyroid. 2001;11(5):501-510. doi:10.1089/105072501300176462

81. Soliman AT, De Sanctis V, Yassin M, Wagdy M, Soliman N. Chronic anemia and thyroid function. Acta Biomed. 2017;88(1):119-127. Published 2017 Apr 28. doi:10.23750/abm.v88i1.6048

82. Walter PB, Knutson MD, Paler-Martinez A, et al. Iron deficiency and iron excess damage mitochondria and mitochondrial DNA in rats. Proc Natl Acad Sci U S A. 2002;99(4):2264-2269. doi:10.1073/pnas.261708798

83. Ness-Abramof R1, Nabriski DA, Prevalence and evaluation of B12 deficiency in patients with autoimmune thyroid disease.Am J Med Sci. 2006 Sep;332(3):119-22.

84. Wang YP, Lin HP. Hemoglobin, iron, and vitamin B12 deficiencies and high blood homocysteine levels in patients with anti-thyroid autoantibodies.J Formos Med Assoc. 2014 Mar;113(3):155-60. doi: 10.1016/j.jfma.2012.04.003. Epub 2012 Jun 29.

85. Jaya Kumari S, Bantwal G Evaluation of serum vitamin B12 levels and its correlation with anti-thyroperoxidase antibody in patients with autoimmune thyroid disorders.Indian J Clin Biochem. 2015 Apr;30(2):217-20. doi: 10.1007/s12291-014-0418-4. Epub 2014 Feb 6.

86. Velarde-Mayol Cl, de la Hoz-García B. Pernicious anemia and autoimmune thyroid diseases in elderly people. Rev Esp Geriatr Gerontol. 2015 May-Jun;50(3):126-8. doi: 10.1016/j.regg.2014.10.004. Epub 2015 Jan 8.

87. Bensky MJ, Ayalon-Dangur I. Comparison of sublingual vs. intramuscular administration of vitamin B12 for the treatment of patients with vitamin B12 deficiency.. Drug Deliv Transl Res. 2019 Jun;9(3):625-630. doi: 10.1007/s13346-018-00613-y.

88. Depeint F, Bruce WR, Shangari N, Mehta R, O'Brien PJ. Mitochondrial function and toxicity: role of B vitamins on the one-carbon transfer pathways. Chem Biol Interact. 2006;163(1-2):113-132. doi:10.1016/j.cbi.2006.05.010

89. Kucharská J. (2008) Vitamins in Mitochondrial Function. In: Gvozdjáková A. (eds) Mitochondrial Medicine. Springer, Dordrecht.

90. Mackawy AM, Al-Ayed BM, Al-Rashidi BM. Vitamin d deficiency and its association with thyroid disease. Int J Health Sci (Qassim). 2013;7(3):267-275. doi:10.12816/0006054

91. Kim D. The Role of Vitamin D in Thyroid Diseases. Int J Mol Sci. 2017;18(9):1949. Published 2017 Sep 12. doi:10.3390/ijms18091949

92. Dzik KP, Skrobot W, Kaczor KB, et al. x Oxid Med Cell Longev. 2019;2019:6835341. Published 2019 Jun 2. doi:10.1155/2019/6835341

93. Wang K, Wei H, Zhang W, Li Z, Ding L, Yu T, Tan L, Liu Y, Liu T, Wang H, Fan Y, Zhang P, Shan Z, Zhu M. Severely low serum magnesium is associated with increased risks of positive anti-thyroglobulin antibody and hypothyroidism: A cross-sectional study. Sci Rep. 2018 Jul 2;8(1):9904. doi: 10.1038/s41598-018-28362-5. PMID: 29967483; PMCID: PMC6028657.

94. Ihnatowicz P, Drywień M, Wątor P, Wojsiat J. The importance of nutritional factors and dietary management of Hashimoto's thyroiditis. Ann Agric Environ Med. 2020 Jun 19;27(2):184-193. doi: 10.26444/aaem/112331. Epub 2019 Oct 2. PMID: 32588591.

95. Yamanaka R, Tabata S, Shindo Y, et al. Mitochondrial Mg(2+) homeostasis decides cellular energy metabolism and vulnerability to stress. Sci Rep. 2016;6:30027. Published 2016 Jul 26. doi:10.1038/srep30027

96. Pilchova I, Klacanova K, Tatarkova Z, Kaplan P, Racay P. The Involvement of Mg2+ in Regulation of Cellular and Mitochondrial Functions. Oxid Med Cell Longev. 2017;2017:6797460. doi:10.1155/2017/6797460

97. Moncayo R, Moncayo H. The WOMED model of benign thyroid disease: Acquired magnesium deficiency due to physical and psychological stressors relates to dysfunction of oxidative phosphorylation. BBA Clin. 2014;3:44-64. Published 2014 Nov 12. doi:10.1016/j.bbacli.2014.11.002\

98. Benvenga S, Ferrari SM, Elia G, et al. Nutraceuticals in Thyroidology: A Review of in Vitro, and in Vivo Animal Studies. Nutrients. 2020;12(5):1337. Published 2020 May 8. doi:10.3390/nu12051337

99. Abd Allah ES, Gomaa AM, Sayed MM. The effect of omega-3 on cognition in hypothyroid adult male rats. Acta Physiol Hung. 2014 Sep;101(3):362-76. doi: 10.1556/APhysiol.101.2014.3.11. PMID: 25183510.

100. Moncayo R, Moncayo H. Applying a systems approach to thyroid physiology: Looking at the whole with a mitochondrial perspective instead of judging single TSH values or why we should know more about mitochondria to understand metabolism. BBA Clin. 2017 Apr 4;7:127-140. doi: 10.1016/j.bbacli.2017.03.004. PMID: 28417080; PMCID: PMC5390562.

101. Quinzii CM, Hirano M. Coenzyme Q and mitochondrial disease. Dev Disabil Res Rev. 2010;16(2):183-188. doi:10.1002/ddrr.108

102. Saini R. Coenzyme Q10: The essential nutrient. J Pharm Bioallied Sci. 2011;3(3):466-467. doi:10.4103/0975-7406.84471

103. An JH, Kim YJ, Kim KJ, Kim SH, Kim NH, Kim HY, Kim NH, Choi KM, Baik SH, Choi DS, Kim SG. L-carnitine supplementation for the management of fatigue in patients with hypothyroidism on levothyroxine treatment: a randomized, double-blind, placebo-controlled trial. Endocr J. 2016 Oct 29;63(10):885-895. doi: 10.1507/endocrj.EJ16-0109. Epub 2016 Jul 16. PMID: 27432821.

104. Benvenga S, Feldt-Rasmussen U, Bonofiglio D, Asamoah E. Nutraceutical Supplements in the Thyroid Setting: Health Benefits beyond Basic Nutrition. Nutrients. 2019 Sep 13;11(9):2214. doi: 10.3390/nu11092214. PMID: 31540254; PMCID: PMC6770945.

105. Sinclair C, Gilchrist, J, Hennessey J, et al. Muscle carnitine in hypo- and hyperthyroidism. Muscle & Nerve. 2005. 32. 357-9. https://www.researchgate.net/publication/7933618_Muscle_carnitine_in_hypo-_and_hyperthyroidism

106. Moncayo R, Moncayo H. Applying a systems approach to thyroid physiology: Looking at the whole with a mitochondrial perspective instead of judging single TSH values or why we should know more about mitochondria to understand metabolism. BBA Clin. 2017 Apr 4; 7:127-140.

107. An JH, Kim YJ, Kim KJ, et al. L-carnitine supplementation for the management of fatigue in patients with hypothyroidism on levothyroxine treatment: a randomized, double-blind, placebo-controlled trial. Endocr J. 2016 Oct 29;63(10):885-895. Epub 2016 Jul 16.

108. Benvenga S, Feldt-Rasmussen U, Bonofiglio D, et al. Nutraceutical supplements in the thyroid setting: health benefits beyond basic nutrition. Nutrients. 2019 Sep 13;11(9). pii: E2214.

109. Samadi Noshahr Z, Shahraki MR, Ahmadvand H, Nourabadi D, Nakhaei A. Protective effects of Withania somnifera root on inflammatory markers and insulin resistance in fructose-fed rats. Rep Biochem Mol Biol. 2015 Apr;3(2):62-7. PMID: 26989739; PMCID: PMC4757043.

110. José M. Zubeldia, Hani A. Nabi. Exploring New Applications for Rhodiola rosea: Can We Improve the Quality of Life of Patients with Short-Term Hypothyroidism Induced by Hormone Withdrawal?. Journal of Medicinal Food 2010 13:6, 1287-1292

111. Kar A, Panda S, Bharti S. Relative efficacy of three medicinal plant extracts in the alteration of thyroid hormone concentrations in male mice. J Ethnopharmacol. 2002 Jul;81(2):281-5. doi: 10.1016/s0378-8741(02)00048-x. PMID: 12065164.

112. Sears ME, Kerr KJ, Bray RI. Arsenic, cadmium, lead, and mercury in sweat: a systematic review. J Environ Public Health. 2012;2012:184745. doi: 10.1155/2012/184745. Epub 2012 Feb 22. PMID: 22505948; PMCID: PMC3312275.

113. Genuis SJ, Beesoon S, Birkholz D, Lobo RA. Human excretion of bisphenol A: blood, urine, and sweat (BUS) study. J Environ Public Health. 2012;2012:185731. doi: 10.1155/2012/185731. Epub 2011 Dec 27. PMID: 22253637; PMCID: PMC3255175.

114. Genuis SJ, Beesoon S, Lobo RA, Birkholz D. Human elimination of phthalate compounds: blood, urine, and sweat (BUS) study. ScientificWorldJournal. 2012;2012:615068. doi: 10.1100/2012/615068. Epub 2012 Oct 31. PMID: 23213291; PMCID: PMC3504417.

115. Vidart J, Wajner SM, Schaan BD, Maia AL. Effect of N-acetylcysteine on serum thyroid hormone levels in nonthyroidal illness

syndrome. Crit Care. 2013;17(Suppl 3): P37. doi:10.1186/cc12653

116. Wright DJ, Renoir T, Smith ZM, et al. N-Acetylcysteine improves mitochondrial function and ameliorates behavioral deficits in the R6/1 mouse model of Huntington's disease. Transl Psychiatry. 2015;5(1): e492. Published 2015 Jan 6. doi:10.1038/tp.2014.13

117. Ladas EJ, Kroll DJ, Oberlies NH, et al. A randomized, controlled, double-blind, pilot study of milk thistle for the treatment of hepatotoxicity in childhood acute lymphoblastic leukemia (ALL). Cancer. 2010;116(2):506-513. doi:10.1002/cncr.24723

118. Li Y, Ma QG, Zhao LH, et al. Effects of lipoic acid on immune function, the antioxidant defense system, and inflammation-related genes expression of broiler chickens fed aflatoxin contaminated diets. Int J Mol Sci. 2014;15(4):5649-5662. Published 2014 Apr 2. doi:10.3390/ijms15045649

119. Patrick L. Mercury toxicity and antioxidants: Part 1: role of glutathione and alpha-lipoic acid in the treatment of mercury toxicity. Altern Med Rev. 2002 Dec;7(6):456-71. PMID: 12495372.

120. Gurer H, Ozgunes H, Oztezcan S, Ercal N. Antioxidant role of alpha-lipoic acid in lead toxicity. Free Radic Biol Med. 1999 Jul;27(1-2):75-81. doi: 10.1016/s0891-5849(99)00036-2. PMID: 10443922.

121. Samanta L, Panigrahi J, Bhanja S, Chainy GB. Effect of turmeric and its active principle curcumin on t(3)-induced oxidative stress and hyperplasia in rat kidney: a comparison. Indian J Clin Biochem. 2010;25(4):393-397. doi:10.1007/s12291-010-0046-6

122. Abdelaleem MM, El-Tahawy NFG, Abozaid SMM, Abdel-Hakim SA. Possible protective effect of curcumin on the thyroid gland changes induced by sodium fluoride in albino rats:

light and electron microscopic study. Endocr Regul. 2018 Apr 1;52(2):59-68. doi: 10.2478/enr-2018-0007. PMID: 29715188.

123. Abd El-Twab, Sanaa M., and Manal Abdul-Hamid. "Curcumin mitigates lithium-induced thyroid dysfunction by modulating antioxidant status, apoptosis and inflammatory cytokines." The Journal of Basic & Applied Zoology 76 (2016): 7-19.

124. Bright JJ. Curcumin and autoimmune disease. Adv Exp Med Biol. 2007;595:425-51. doi: 10.1007/978-0-387-46401-5_19. PMID: 17569223.

125. Mishra P, Paital B, Jena S, Swain SS, Kumar S, Yadav MK, Chainy GBN, Samanta L. Possible activation of NRF2 by Vitamin E/Curcumin against altered thyroid hormone induced oxidative stress via NFκB/AKT/mTOR/KEAP1 signalling in rat heart. Sci Rep. 2019 May 15;9(1):7408. doi: 10.1038/s41598-019-43320-5. PMID: 31092832; PMCID: PMC6520394.

126. Lara Gibellini, Elena Bianchini, Sara De Biasi, Milena Nasi, Andrea Cossarizza, Marcello Pinti, "Natural Compounds Modulating Mitochondrial Functions", Evidence-Based Complementary and Alternative Medicine, vol. 2015, Article ID 527209, 13 pages, 2015. https://doi.org/10.1155/2015/527209

127. Bagheri, Hossein & Ghasemi, Faezeh & Barreto, George & Rafiee, Rouhullah & Sathyapalan, Thozhukat & Sahebkar, Amirhossein. (2019). Effects of curcumin on mitochondria in neurodegenerative diseases. BioFactors. 46. 10.1002/biof.1566.

128. de Oliveira MR, Jardim FR, Setzer WN, Nabavi SM, Nabavi SF. Curcumin, mitochondrial biogenesis, and mitophagy: Exploring recent data and indicating future needs. Biotechnol Adv. 2016 Sep-Oct;34(5):813-826. doi: 10.1016/j.biotechadv.2016.04.004. Epub 2016 May 1. PMID: 27143655.

129. 129. The PSS Scale of the American Sociological Association, from Cohen, S., Kamarck, T., and Mermelstein, R. (1983). A

global measure of perceived stress. Journal of Health and Social Behavior, 24,386-396.

130. 130. Cohen, S. and Williamson, G. Perceived Stress in a Probability Sample of the United States. Spacapan, S. and Oskamp, S. (Eds.) TheSocial Psychology of Health.Newbury Park, CA: Sage, 1988.

Made in United States
Troutdale, OR
02/29/2024